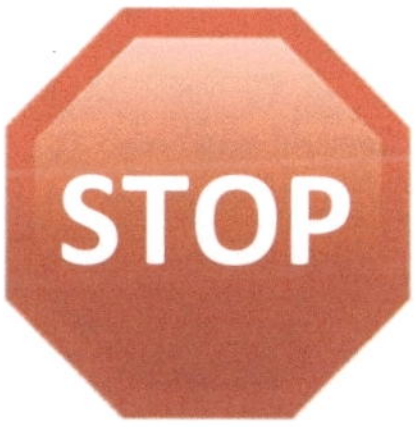

FREE COURSE VIDEO!

The purchase of each new copy of *After Ablation* includes online access to a free course video. To receive free access to the course, email **course@rxstudyguides.com** with "FREE COURSE" in the subject line. In the body of the email, include your full name and a screenshot of your receipt/proof of purchase indicating that you purchased a new copy of the book.

Upon receiving your email, we'll send you instructions on accessing the online course video.

Kind regards,

David Heckman, PharmD Author of After Ablation

AFTER ABLATION

PREVENTING ATRIAL FIBRILLATION RECURRENCE
WITH INSIGHTS FROM OVER 120 RESEARCH PAPERS

BY DAVID HECKMAN, PHARMD

After Ablation: Preventing Atrial Fibrillation Recurrence with Insights from Over 120 Research Papers

ISBN-13: 978-1-942682-18-9

Published by David Heckman, PharmD

THE GOAL

To prevent the recurrence of atrial fibrillation after a successful ablation.

THE CONCEPT

Atrial fibrillation (AF) is a progressive and often debilitating disease. AF increases the probability of stroke by up to 5X and death by roughly 2X.[10-13] Around 35% of those with AF suffer from severe anxiety and distress, and 20% have reported suicidal thoughts.[19] While cardiac catheter ablation offers the possibility of long-term freedom from AF, a high percentage of those receiving an ablation experience AF recurrence within a few years. Few studies have investigated the prevention of AF recurrence *after ablation*. Yet, those who recently received an ablation are among the most motivated to make the lifestyle changes necessary to reduce AF risk. Much of the research in this area explores 1) how various factors might impact the development of AF in populations with no history of arrhythmia or 2) how specific interventions might reduce the frequency and duration of AF episodes in patients with an active AF diagnosis. In the absence of more targeted research, we can reasonably borrow what has been gleaned from this less targeted research and employ it to prevent AF recurrences *after ablation*. Though imperfect, the merit of attempting to prevent arrhythmia recurrences outweighs the alternative, which is to do nothing.

THE EVIDENCE

In the ARREST-AF trial, the authors (Pathak et al.) suggest AF recurrences after ablation "may be due to failure to attenuate the progressive substrate promoted by cardiovascular risk factors."[20] Their clinical trial demonstrated that 87% of patients participating in a risk factor management program after ablation experienced continued freedom from AF at their final follow-up visit (average follow-up period of 3.5 years) compared to only 18% of those who did not participate in the risk factor management program.[20]

18%

Ablation success rate with
traditional medical treatment only

87%

Ablation success rate with
traditional medical treatment
+ risk factor management

STATEMENT FROM THE AMERICAN HEART ASSOCIATION (2020):

"...emerging evidence supports that addressing these modifiable risks may be effective for primary and secondary AF prevention. A structured, protocol-driven multidisciplinary approach to integrate lifestyle and risk factor management as an integral part of AF management may help in the prevention and treatment of AF. However, this aspect of AF management is currently underrecognized, underused, and understudied."[21]

THE COMPLEXITY
of ATRIAL FIBRILLATION

The following have been implicated in the development and perpetuation of atrial fibrillation (AF):

✓Physical inactivity ✓Participation in extreme endurance athletics ✓Emotional and psychological stress
✓Anger ✓Hostility ✓Depression ✓Anxiety ✓Panic disorder ✓Tension ✓Job strain
✓Night shift work ✓Sleep deprivation ✓Obstructive sleep apnea ✓Overweight ✓Obesity
✓Alcohol ✓Cigarette smoking ✓High blood pressure ✓High triglycerides
✓Low HDL cholesterol ✓Oxidative stress ✓Atrial fibrosis
✓Atrial stretching ✓Heart failure ✓Heart valve disease
✓Coronary heart disease
✓Inflammation

Despite this complexity, healthcare providers must–as a matter of practical and economic necessity–treat AF like any other disease... with systematic efficiency, relying on quick, high-impact interventions (i.e., prescription drugs and surgical procedures). Unfortunately, however, medications and ablations often fail to provide long-term freedom from AF. Given the glut of factors implicated in the development of AF, it is not surprising that recent research suggests a more holistic approach might produce dramatically better results.

"Nearly 60% of atrial fibrillation (AF) can be attributed to modifiable risk factors."

"Because there is no cure for AF and patients are forced to manage AF as a chronic disease, prevention of AF is the optimal approach..."

- Heart. 2017 Aug;103(15):1141-1142.

"Specific interventions aimed at controlling risk factors have been [shown] to clearly reduce the risk of AF in several cohorts."

"Even more importantly, integrated [programs] aimed at controlling for multiple risk factors would be more efficient in terms of reducing risk of AF..."

"Indeed, several studies recently published point out how targeted interventions could be useful in reducing the risk of AF occurrence (or recurrence)."

- Heart. 2018 Jun;104(11):882-887.

"...therapy targeting risk factors and underlying conditions is an emerging AF management strategy that warrants better implementation in clinical practice."

- Arrhythm Electrophysiol Rev. 2018 Jun;7(2):118-127.

"...more recently, risk factor management has gained significant momentum."

"Targeting underlying predisposing conditions that are associated with the development and progression of AF seems prudent."

- J Arrhythm. 2019 Nov 6;35(6):781-788.

"Comprehensive management of cardiovascular risk factors has been associated with the greatest likelihood of freedom from arrhythmia recurrence post-ablation."

- J Clin Med. 2022 May 9;11(9):2660.

THE METHOD & RATIONALE

Risk factor management program protocols from the LEGACY and ARREST-AF trials should serve as the backbone of an evidence-based strategy to prevent AF recurrences after ablation. This book builds on that foundation by outlining several tweaks and additional research-based interventions that could be included as part of an individualized AF recurrence prevention strategy.

The risk factor management program employed in the ARREST-AF trial produced a long-term ablation success rate of 87%. Why even attempt to improve upon this achievement? As with any clinical trial, feasibility constrains trial design. In other words, clinical trial protocols must be relatively cheap and convenient to execute as a matter of practical and economic necessity. The beauty of writing a book like this is that there are no constraints. We need not limit ourselves to any number of targets and goals. On the contrary, we can include as many targets and goals as the research findings can support.

PROCEED WITH CAUTION

In theory/when possible, medical interventions are based on evidence ("evidence-based medicine"). Broadly, we can say that medical evidence comes from six types of published research,[22] and the rank order of the quality/strength of the findings produced by said research is as follows[23]:

Top of the medical evidence hierarchy
↓
#1 Meta-Analyses and Systematic Reviews
> #2 Randomized Controlled Trials > #3 Cohort Studies
> #4 Case-Control Studies > #5 Cross Sectional Surveys > #6 Case Reports

Many people view published research findings as factual until proven otherwise, predicated on the assumption that the research has been conducted honestly. Consider this. Physician and self-taught statistician David Carlisle found that among 526 clinical trials submitted to a medical journal for publication, around 20% contained falsified or fabricated data.[24] John Ioannidis, Professor of Medicine at Stanford University and author of the famous article "Why Most Published Research Findings Are False," estimates that up to 90% of published medical research is flawed.[25] One factor contributing to this problem is publication bias. Clinical trials with positive findings are almost four times more likely to be published than trials with negative or null findings.[26] This can have multiple downstream effects, not the least of which is encouraging researchers to manipulate data to produce or strengthen positive findings. Meanwhile, the "evidence" produced by published research forms the entire basis of evidence-based medicine.[27] Other issues affect the integrity of the "evidence" upon which we base our medical decisions; for instance, 58% of biomedical research is funded by corporations.[28] Meanwhile, industry-funded research is about two times more likely than non-industry-funded research to generate results that favor the new industry product.[29]

Even in a world void of bias and dishonesty, we would expect to stumble slowly toward the truth in a fashion similar to that depicted below, where each black dot represents a clinical study.

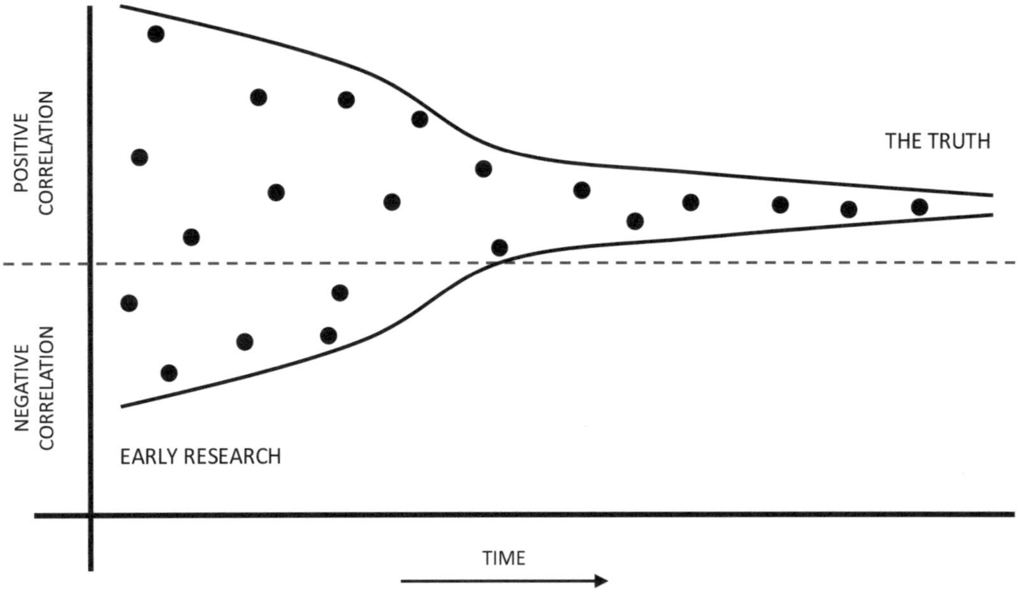

All this to say, some of the interventions outlined in this book are based on early research. While taking the risk of highlighting information based on the findings of early research, the author has attempted to limit the review of potentially helpful interventions to include only those estimated to have an excellent safety profile. When safety concerns exist, the author has attempted to provide appropriate warnings. As a reminder, this book does not constitute medical advice.

PROCEED WITH CAUTION

To illustrate the danger of drawing conclusions based on the findings of early research, consider chocolate and omega-3 fatty acids. Years ago, some doctors recommended chocolate consumption and omega-3 fatty acid supplementation to lower AF risk. However, now it is relatively clear that chocolate consumption does not reduce AF risk, and omega-3 fatty acid supplementation may increase AF risk. So why were some doctors willing to tout early research findings and risk harming their patients in the long run? Perhaps because they believed any risks associated with routine chocolate consumption or omega-3 fatty acid supplementation would be negligible. In the case of chocolate consumption, they would have been correct. Unfortunately, however, omega-3 fatty acid supplements do not appear to be so harmless.

A REVIEW OF CURRENT EVIDENCE ON CHOCOLATE AND AF RISK

A 2018 meta-analysis of five cohort studies revealed that chocolate consumption does not influence the risk of AF.[30] Given the importance of achieving and maintaining a BMI < 25 kg/m^2, the routine consumption of chocolate for the remote possibility of a slight reduction in AF risk might be negated in the long run by its negative impact on body weight/body composition.

A REVIEW OF CURRENT EVIDENCE ON OMEGA-3 FATTY ACIDS AND AF RISK

Recent data suggest the more EPA/DHA a person consumes from supplements, the more likely they are to develop AF. This was demonstrated by a randomized control trial published in 2020. During the 3 ½-year study period, AF was 69% more likely in the omega-3 fatty acid group (4 grams/day) compared to the placebo control group.[31] Further evidence against EPA and DHA came from a randomized controlled trial published in 2021. During the 5-year study period, AF was 9% more likely to occur in the group receiving omega-3 fatty acids (840 mg of EPA/DHA per day) than in the placebo group.[32] This finding suggests that even low doses (< 1 gram/day) may contribute to the development of AF.

#1
BODYWEIGHT

BODYWEIGHT

"Obesity begets atrial fibrillation."[33]

"Obesity has been estimated to account for one-fifth of all AF..."[34]

Each one-unit increase in body mass index (BMI) is associated with a 3-8% higher risk of developing AF.[34-36]

One year after ablation, AF recurrence is 20% more likely to occur in those who are obese (BMI ≥ 30 kg/m^2) compared to those who are overweight (BMI 25.5–29 kg/m^2).[37]

WEIGHT LOSS & ATRIAL FIBRILLATION

≥ 10% WEIGHT LOSS	3–9% WEIGHT LOSS	< 3% WEIGHT LOSS
★ **45.5%** ★	**22.2%**	**13.4%**
Probability of long-term freedom from AF[4]	Probability of long-term freedom from AF[4]	Probability of long-term freedom from AF[4]

Note the average participant in this study was obese (average BMI of approximately 33 kg/m^2), and no one in these groups received antiarrhythmic medication or catheter ablation; however, participants concurrently addressed other AF/cardiac risk factors (alcohol consumption, high blood pressure, high blood sugar, high cholesterol, sleep apnea, and smoking).

HOW TO LOSE WEIGHT

Most people have strong opinions on weight loss and nutrition. However, regardless of personal opinion, research has proven that weight loss occurs as a consequence of a calorie deficit.[38] Furthermore, "reduced-calorie diets result in clinically meaningful weight loss regardless of which macronutrients they emphasize."[39] This should be achieved through long-term modification of dietary intake and increased physical activity.

WEIGHT FLUCTUATIONS

A weight fluctuation greater than 5% (with one year between measurements) doubles the risk of AF onset/recurrence.[4,40] Note that a "weight fluctuation" is defined as a loss followed by a gain or a gain followed by a loss. For this reason, it is critical to maintain the new body weight.

EXCESS WEIGHT & INFLAMMATION

In the research that laid the foundation for this book (the LEGACY and ARREST-AF trials), researchers monitored participants' high-sensitivity C-reactive protein (hs-CRP) levels, highlighting the importance of inflammation in the development of AF. The presence of inflammation in the heart (or throughout the body) predicts the onset/recurrence of AF. Furthermore, high levels of inflammation have been associated with ischemic strokes, perhaps the most feared complication of AF.[41] Logic follows that any strategy designed to prevent AF should include measures to combat inflammation. According to the lifestyle inflammation scores developed by Byrd et al. (see page 15), being overweight or obese triggers more inflammation than any other factor assessed.[42]

★ WEIGHT MANAGEMENT PROGRAM ★

As demonstrated in multiple studies, participation in a structured weight management program is critical to long-term ablation success.[4,20,43]

#2 MEAL PLANNING

MEAL PLANNING

In the LEGACY and ARREST-AF trials, meals were planned to include high-protein, low glycemic index, calorie-controlled foods. However, at the time of this writing, the Mediterranean diet (MedDiet) has the most substantial evidence of any eating pattern for preventing AF. Therefore, the MedDiet should be the preferred (until further notice) lifelong diet of choice for anyone attempting to minimize their risk of developing new or recurrent AF. Fortunately, the benefits of the MedDiet extend far beyond AF risk reduction. To illustrate this point, we look to the results of the landmark clinical trial, PREDIMED.

The PREDIMED trial represents "the largest primary prevention trial ever testing the effects of changes in a complete food pattern (namely, the Mediterranean diet) on cardiovascular disease."[44]

The PREDIMED trial (conducted 2003-2010) compared three diets (the Mediterranean diet with mixed nuts, the Mediterranean diet with extra-virgin olive oil (EVOO), and a low-fat diet) in 7,447 Spanish patients who were at high risk for developing cardiovascular disease. No calorie restriction was advised, nor was exercise promoted.[45] The Mediterranean diet (MedDiet) was associated with the following relative risk reductions (compared to a low-fat diet):

Disease	**MedDiet with mixed nuts**	**MedDiet with EVOO**
Atrial fibrillation[46]	↓11%	↓38%
Heart attack, stroke, and death from cardiovascular causes[45]	↓28%	↓31%
Type II diabetes[47]	↓18%	↓40%
Peripheral arterial disease[48]	↓50%	↓66%
Breast cancer[49]	↓47%	↓69%
Heart failure[50]	↓8%	↓32%

Guided by the results of the PREDIMED trial, we can cautiously conclude that the Mediterranean diet supplemented with EVOO is the healthiest dietary pattern, not only for the prevention of AF but also for the prevention of many other diseases. What makes EVOO so unique probably has something to do with the fact that it contains more than 200 chemical compounds, including both water- and fat-soluble phenols.[51]

TOP 5 PRINCIPLES OF THE MEDITERRANEAN DIET FROM THE PREDIMED TRIAL PROTOCOL

#1 High consumption of whole grains, legumes, nuts, vegetables, and fruits

#2 Relatively high fat consumption, primarily from EVOO in cooking and dressing of vegetables

#3 Moderate to high consumption of fish

#4 Moderate to low consumption of poultry and dairy products (usually in the form of yogurt or cheese)

#5 Low consumption of red meat and processed meat

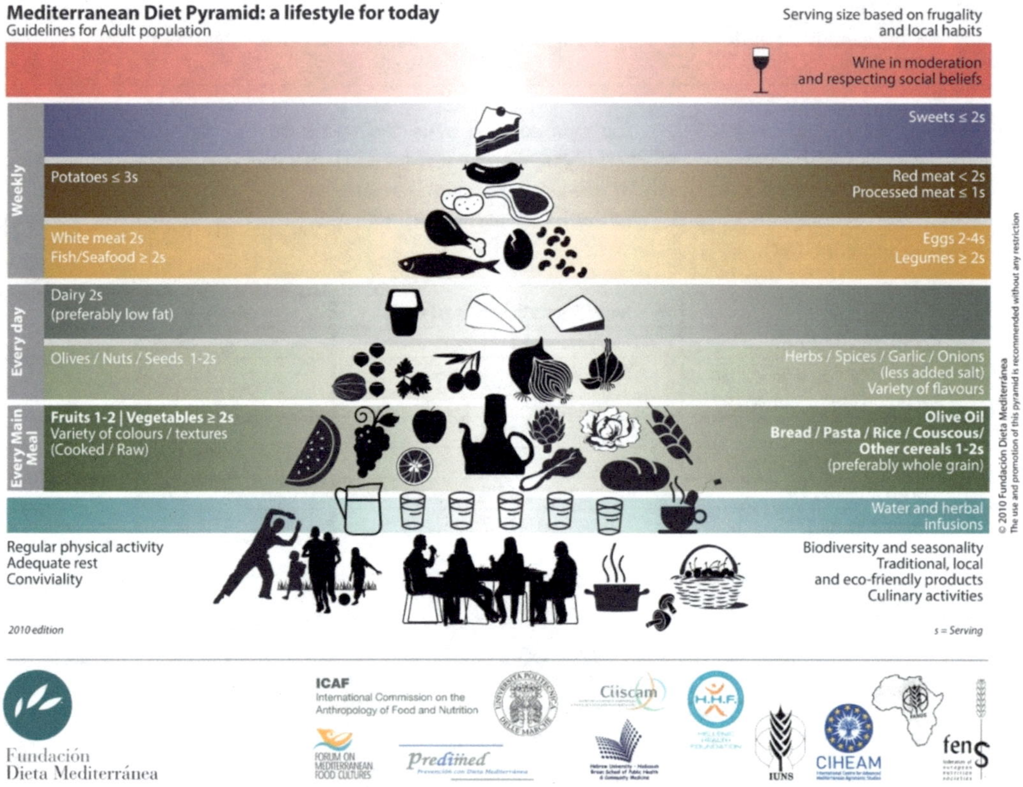

Source: Bach-Faig A, Berry EM, Lairon D, et al. Mediterranean diet pyramid today. Science and cultural updates. Public Health Nutr. 2011;14(12A):2274-2284. doi:10.1017/S1368980011002515

INFLAMMATORY IMPACT
OF LIFESTYLE FACTORS AND FOODS/BEVERAGES

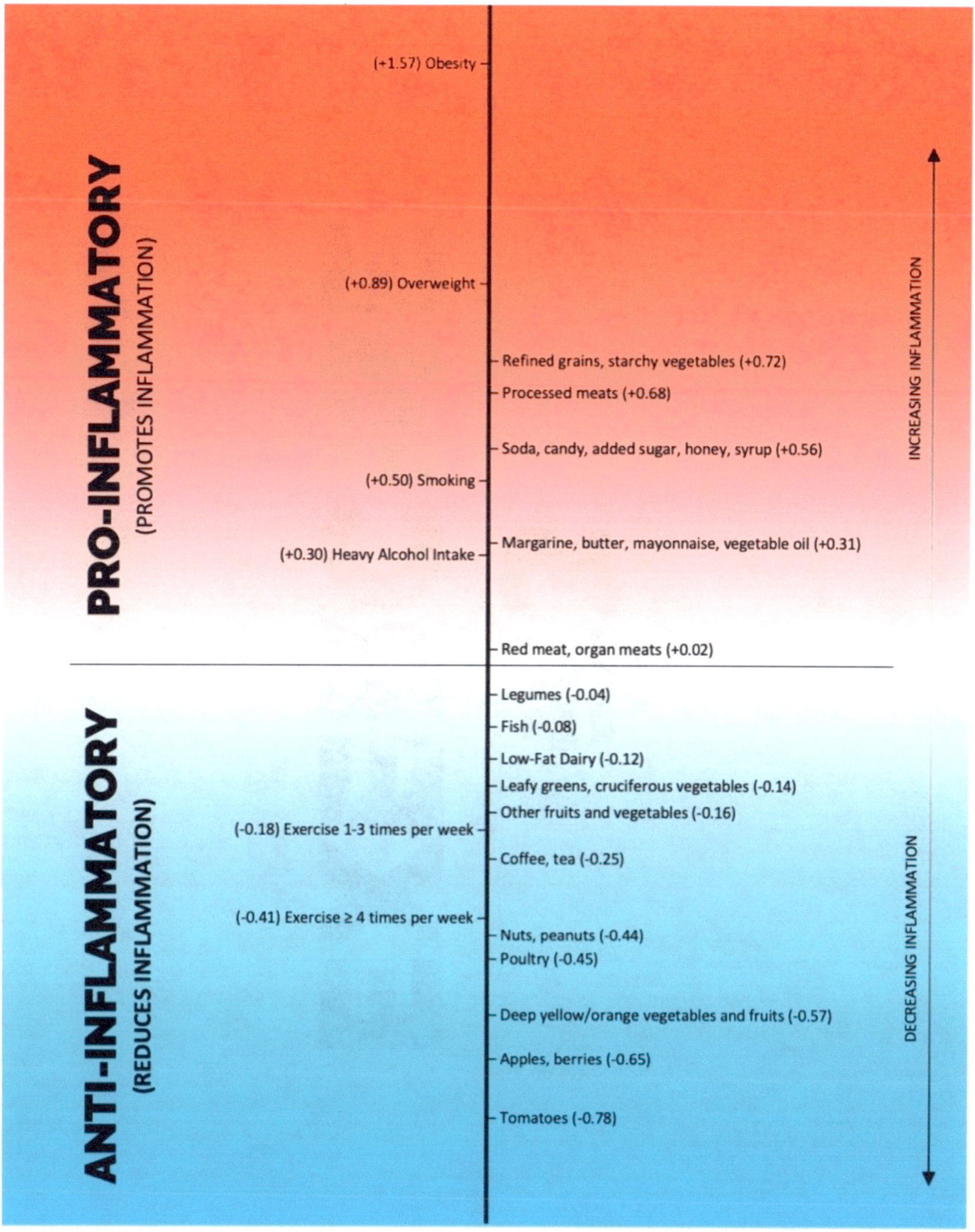

Illustration based on data from Byrd DA, Judd SE, Flanders WD, Hartman TJ, Fedirko V, Bostick RM. Development and Validation of Novel Dietary and Lifestyle Inflammation Scores. J Nutr. 2019;149(12):2206-2218.

#3
EXERCISE

EXERCISE

Regular physical activity + high cardiorespiratory fitness = ↓risk of atrial fibrillation[52]

"Indeed, emerging research has demonstrated beneficial effects of exercise on AF-specific outcomes, including AF recurrence post-ablation."[18]

PHYSICAL ACTIVITY

In most published research examining associations between physical activity and AF, researchers acquired physical activity data exclusively from self-reported questionnaires.[9] That's a big problem. The typical person does an abysmal job of accurately self-reporting physical activity.[53] More recently, scientists studying this issue have employed modern wearable technologies (i.e., smartwatches with accelerometers) to measure physical activity objectively. Below is a broad-strokes representation of the findings of one such study from 2021 that included more than 93,00 participants. The illustrations on the next page provide a more detailed breakdown of the data.

175-220 MINUTES/WEEK

Compared to 0-20 minutes/week, 175-220 minutes/week of moderate to vigorous physical activity was associated with a 41% reduction in AF risk and a 49% reduction in stroke risk.[54]

PROBABILITY OF AF

↓41%

PROBABILITY OF STROKE

↓49%

While some of the AF-protective effects of exercise appear to be lost with larger volumes of moderate to vigorous physical activity (> 395 minutes/week), the risk of stroke was reduced by an additional 3%. This illustrates a broader point about high-volume physical activity–although it may increase AF risk, it is associated with a lower overall risk of death.

EXERCISE: A POTENT ANTI-INFLAMMATORY

According to the lifestyle inflammation scores developed by Byrd et al. (see page 15), exercising four or more times per week produces the most potent anti-inflammatory effect of all lifestyle factors assessed.[42]

RISK OF ATRIAL FIBRILLATION

BASED ON TIME IN MODERATE TO VIGOROUS PHYSICAL ACTIVITY

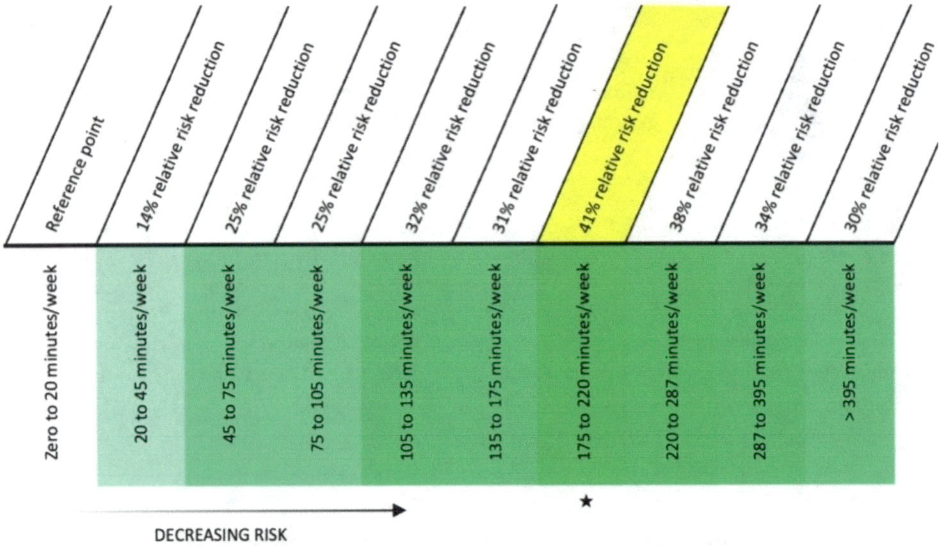

Data from Khurshid S, Weng LC, Al-Alusi MA, et al. Accelerometer-derived physical activity and risk of atrial fibrillation. Eur Heart J. 2021;42(25 Suppl):S13.

RISK OF STROKE

BASED ON TIME IN MODERATE TO VIGOROUS PHYSICAL ACTIVITY

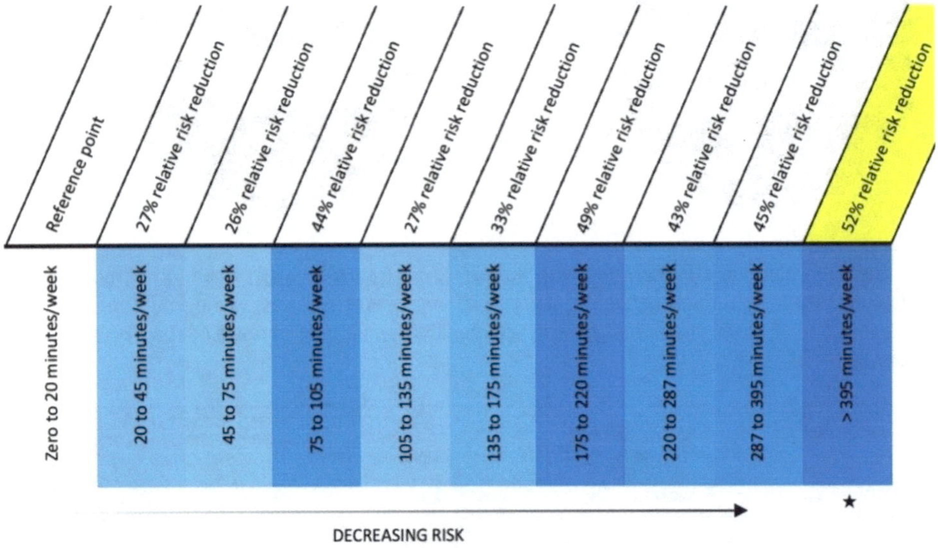

Data from Khurshid S, Weng LC, Al-Alusi MA, et al. Accelerometer-derived physical activity and risk of atrial fibrillation. Eur Heart J. 2021;42(25 Suppl):S13.

MODERATE VERSUS VIGOROUS PHYSICAL ACTIVITY

According to this study, the optimal volume of moderate to vigorous physical activity is 175-220 minutes/week. However, other research suggests high volume vigorous physical activity (particularly for men) increases AF risk.

> "Extreme endurance training produces structural and functional cardiac adaptations, higher levels of oxidative stress, inflammation, and adrenergic activation, ultimately predisposing to atrial fibrosis and AF."[8]

> "...although vigorous exercise may be associated with increased AF risk, moderate physical activity is protective."[14]

Therefore, should one limit participation in vigorous physical activity? According to one study, participants who achieved 28-40 minutes per week of vigorous physical activity (and spent the remaining time performing moderate physical activity) enjoyed the most significant reduction in AF risk.[54] However, this is just one study. More research is needed to clarify "the amount, intensity, and duration of physical activity beyond which the risk of AF increases."[9]

In 2021, a large meta-analysis of 23 studies (involving more than 1.9 million participants) was published in the European Journal of Epidemiology. The authors' opinion on this topic is presented below.

> "The evidence on the vascular health and mortality benefits attributed to regular physical activity is overwhelming. Even for high-intensity (i.e., vigorous) physical activity regimens whose intensities and volumes far exceed those proposed by guideline recommendations, their long-term protective effects on mortality by far outweigh their risk of adverse events such as AF."[9]

Meanwhile, other experts take a more conservative stance.

> "...we advocate regular (but not long-term high-intensity endurance) exercise training as a safe and effective strategy to reduce the risk of incident AF and to minimize the associated risk of secondary cardiovascular events."[18]

METABOLIC EQUIVALENT TASKS (METs)

"One MET is defined as the amount of oxygen consumed while sitting at rest... The MET concept represents a simple, practical, and easily understood procedure for expressing the energy cost of physical activities as a multiple of the resting metabolic rate."[55]

SEDENTARY	LIGHT INTENSITY	MODERATE INTENSITY	VIGOROUS INTENSITY
1.0–1.5 METs	**1.6–3.0 METs**	**3.0–6.0 METs**	**6.0+ METs**
Example: sitting	Example: walking slow	Example: walking fast	Example: running

For a comprehensive list of physical activities and their associated MET values, do a Google search for the "Compendium of Physical Activities."

PRACTICAL INTERPRETATION OF MET VALUES

Many consumer devices estimate calories burned during exercise but do not provide MET estimates. Though the conversion is imperfect, one MET roughly equals a burn rate of one calorie per minute.[56] Therefore, if a person burns 50 calories while cycling on a stationary bike for 10 minutes, they are burning five calories per minute, which is roughly equivalent to 5 METs.

Regular physical activity + high cardiorespiratory fitness = ↓risk of atrial fibrillation[52]

"Higher cardiorespiratory fitness is associated with reduced arrhythmia recurrence rates and death among patients undergoing AF ablation."[5]

HIGH CARDIORESPIRATORY FITNESS	ADEQUATE CARDIORESPIRATORY FITNESS	LOW CARDIORESPIRATORY FITNESS
★ **27.5%** ★	**54%**	**79%**
Probability of AF recurrence within 32 months after ablation[5]	Probability of AF recurrence within 32 months after ablation[5]	Probability of AF recurrence within 32 months after ablation[5]

"High cardiorespiratory fitness" was defined as metabolic equivalent tasks (METs) achieved during treadmill stress test > 100% of predicted, "adequate cardiorespiratory fitness" was defined as 85–100% of predicted, and "low cardiorespiratory fitness" was defined as < 85% of predicted.

CALCULATING PREDICTED CARDIORESPIRATORY FITNESS

In the study referenced above, "predicted cardiorespiratory fitness" was calculated as follows:

♂

MEN

Predicted METs = 18 – (0.15 x age)

♀

WOMEN

Predicted METs = 14.7 – (0.13 x age)

TREADMILL STRESS TEST PROTOCOL

Duration	Speed	Grade/Incline	METs
3 minutes	1.7 mph	10%	4
3 minutes	2.5 mph	12%	7
3 minutes	3.3 mph	14%	10
3 minutes	4.2 mph	16%	13
3 minutes	5.0 mph	18%	16
3 minutes	5.5 mph	20%	18

The treadmill stress test protocol outlined in the table above (known as the Bruce protocol) can be used to determine cardiorespiratory fitness. A treadmill stress test should be conducted under medical supervision. Fortunately, there is a much more manageable, albeit less accurate, alternative. Many devices (e.g., smartwatches, chest strap heart rate sensors) can estimate cardiorespiratory fitness in terms of VO2 max. VO2 max can then be converted to METs using the following conversion factor: 1 MET = 3.5 mL/kg/min.[57]

CONVERTING VO2 MAX TO METs

Imagine we have Bob, a 50-year-old man with an estimated VO2 max of 40 mL/kg/min (VO2 max estimated by smartwatch). How do we express Bob's cardiorespiratory fitness in terms of METs? What is Bob's predicted cardiorespiratory fitness? Based on this information, is Bob's cardiorespiratory fitness high, adequate, or low?

STEP 1: Convert VO2 max to METs.

$$40 \text{ mL/kg/min} \times \frac{1 \text{ MET}}{3.5 \text{ mL/kg/min}} = 11.4 \text{ METs}$$

STEP 2: Calculate "predicted cardiorespiratory fitness" based on the equation for men.

$$\begin{aligned} \text{Predicted METs} &= 18 - (0.15 \times \text{age}) \\ &= 18 - (0.15 \times 50) \\ &= 18 - 7.5 \\ &= 10.5 \end{aligned}$$

STEP 3: Divide the answer from STEP 1 by the answer from STEP 2 to determine the percent of predicted cardiorespiratory fitness achieved.

$$\frac{11.4 \text{ METs}}{10.5 \text{ METs}} = 1.086 \rightarrow 108.6\%$$

∴ Bob's cardiorespiratory fitness level is high (> 100% of predicted).

THE BENEFITS OF SLIGHTLY IMPROVING CARDIORESPIRATORY FITNESS

Each one-MET increase in cardiorespiratory fitness (CRF) is associated with a 10% reduction in the risk of AF recurrence after ablation.[14,33] The benefits of improving CRF are not isolated to AF. In study participants who improved CRF > 1 MET, researchers observed the following additional benefits:

#1 Weight loss #2 Better glycemic control (lower HbA1c levels)
#3 Decreased inflammation (lower hs-CRP levels) #4 Lower LDL cholesterol and triglyceride levels
#5 Lower blood pressure/reduced need for blood pressure medication #6 Reduced left atrial volume

---

#4 BLOOD PRESSURE

BLOOD PRESSURE

HYPERTENSION
73% ↑RISK
of ATRIAL FIBRILLATION

"Patients with hypertension are 73% more likely than those with normal blood pressure levels to develop AF..."[8]

NORMAL BLOOD PRESSURE → less than $\frac{120 \text{ mmHg}}{80 \text{ mmHg}}$

120 mmHg ← systolic blood pressure

80 mmHg ← diastolic blood pressure

Even at systolic blood pressure levels once considered to be "pre-hypertension" or "high normal" (≥ 130 mmHg), the risk of AF is heightened.[14,58]

SALT RESTRICTION

In the LEGACY and ARREST-AF trials, participants were advised to restrict salt intake. Reducing daily salt consumption by 6 grams (1 teaspoon) leads to a roughly 10 mmHg decrease in systolic blood pressure and an estimated 17% decrease in the risk of a stroke.[59]

RESEARCH-BASED BLOOD PRESSURE-LOWERING DIETARY CHANGES

Additional dietary changes are likely to further reduce elevated systolic blood pressure. Three high-impact examples are presented below.

FRUITS & VEGETABLES	HIBISCUS TEA	GARLIC
8-10 servings/day[17]	1 cup with each meal[15]	1-2 cloves/day[1]
↓7.2 mmHg	**↓7.2 mmHg**	**↓6.7 mmHg**

Note: The blood pressure-lowering effect of these dietary interventions is less pronounced for those with normal blood pressure. Limit fresh garlic intake to 4 grams (1 small clove) per day if taking antithrombotic medications (e.g., warfarin, clopidogrel), as larger quantities may increase the risk of bleeding.

ANTI-HYPERTENSIVES PROVEN TO REDUCE THE RISK OF AF RECURRENCE

If medication is needed to lower blood pressure, drugs that inhibit the renin-angiotensin-aldosterone system have been proven to prevent new and recurrent AF. Among the options are angiotensin converting enzyme inhibitors (generic name ends in "–pril") and angiotensin receptor blockers (generic name ends in "–sartan").[8]

#5 BLOOD SUGAR

BLOOD SUGAR

PREDIABETES
20% ↑RISK
of ATRIAL FIBRILLATION[2]

DIABETES
28% ↑RISK
of ATRIAL FIBRILLATION[2]

High blood sugar is a hallmark sign of diabetes and prediabetes. Therefore, the primary goal in treating these conditions is to normalize blood sugar levels. The most common lab tests for monitoring blood sugar are fasting blood glucose and hemoglobin A1c. Fasting blood glucose measures the concentration of sugar (glucose) in the blood after a fasting period of 8-12 hours. Hemoglobin A1c (HbA1c) reflects the average blood sugar level during the preceding 2-3 months.

FASTING BLOOD GLUCOSE

NORMAL	**PREDIABETES**	**DIABETES**
Fasting Blood Glucose	Fasting Blood Glucose	Fasting Blood Glucose
< 100 mg/dL	100–125 mg/dL	≥ 126 mg/dL

Each 20 mg/dL increase in fasting blood glucose increases the risk of developing AF by approximately 11%.[2]

HEMOGLOBIN A1c (HbA1c)

NORMAL	**PREDIABETES**	**DIABETES**
HbA1c ≤ 5.6%	HbA1c 5.7–6.4%	HbA1c ≥ 6.5%

The risk of cardiovascular disease increases by 39% for each 1% increase in HbA1c (e.g., from 5% to 6%).[60]

LIFESTYLE CHANGES AND MEDICATIONS

Fortunately, applying the lifestyle changes outlined previously (weight loss, exercise, meal planning) would benefit blood glucose/HbA1c levels and, in approximately 40% of cases, could even reverse type II diabetes.[61] Furthermore, when medically necessary, anti-diabetic medications (e.g., metformin, sulfonylureas, SGLT-2 inhibitors, DPP-4 inhibitors, GLP-1 agonists, and thiazolidinediones) have been shown to reduce AF risk.[62]

#6 CHOLESTEROL

CHOLESTEROL

In the LEGACY and ARREST-AF trials, researchers targeted LDL cholesterol; however, most currently available data suggest that only low HDL cholesterol and high triglycerides are associated with a heightened risk of atrial fibrillation (AF).[3] At the time of this writing, an association between LDL cholesterol and AF has not been established.

HDL ≥ 60 mg/dL
36% ↓RISK
of* ATRIAL FIBRILLATION

TRIGLYCERIDES ≥200 mg/dL
60% ↑RISK
of* ATRIAL FIBRILLATION*

*Compared to study participants with HDL levels < 40 mg/dL.[3]

**Compared to study participants with triglyceride levels < 150 mg/dL.[3]

HOW TO IMPROVE HDL AND TRIGLYCERIDES

While HDL and triglyceride levels are determined partly by genetics, significant improvements can be achieved simply by applying the lifestyle changes outlined in this book–losing weight, improving diet, exercising regularly, reducing alcohol intake, and stopping smoking.[63,64]

STATINS MAY REDUCE THE RISK OF ATRIAL FIBRILLATION BY 50%

The use of statins (a class of cholesterol-lowering drugs) has been associated with a roughly 50% reduction in the relative risk of AF. Specifically, Lipitor® (atorvastatin) and Zocor® (simvastatin) appear to be the most effective for AF risk reduction.[65] It has been theorized that this benefit is due to the anti-inflammatory effects of statin drugs, as opposed to their cholesterol-lowering effects.

RISKS AND BENEFITS OF STATINS

The use of statins increases the relative risk of developing diabetes by approximately 9%. To quantify this risk in absolute terms, treating 255 patients with a statin for four years would result in one extra case of diabetes."[66] A much more common side effect is myalgia (muscle pain). In the literature, it has been reported that one in 21 patients taking a statin experiences muscle pain.[67] In actuality, the prevalence of muscle pain due to statin use may be much higher. Statins can also interfere with the production of coenzyme Q10 (CoQ10).[68]

The research on statin benefits has demonstrated that 167 patients would need to be treated with a statin for 4.1 years to prevent one death, 77 patients would need to be treated to avoid one major coronary event (e.g., heart attack), and 250 patients would need to be treated to prevent one cerebrovascular event (e.g., stroke).[69] These numbers represent averages based on an analysis of 10 studies involving people *without* established cardiovascular disease. The expected risk-benefit profile varies from individual to individual, and there would likely be more benefit for an individual with established cardiovascular disease.

#7 ALCOHOL

ALCOHOL

8% ↑RISK

***of* ATRIAL FIBRILLATION PER DAILY DRINK *of* ALCOHOL[70]**

"There are no safe recommended levels of alcohol consumption…"[71]
– World Heart Federation

"…alcohol consumption, even at moderate intakes, is a risk factor for AF."[70]

MORE REASONS TO QUIT DRINKING

Alcohol is classified as a human carcinogen.[72]

The lifetime risk of developing alcohol dependence is 12.5%.[73]

Alcohol consumption causes inflammation, fat accumulation, and fibrosis.[74]

Alcohol is estimated to be responsible for 4.5% of global injury and disease burden and 4% of all deaths.[75]

THE MEDITERRANEAN DIET

The traditional Mediterranean diet includes moderate alcohol consumption (mainly red wine). Those wishing to mimic the Mediterranean diet as closely as possible may consider dealcoholized or non-alcoholic wine.

#8
SLEEP APNEA

SLEEP APNEA

2X

After ablation, obstructive sleep apnea roughly doubles the probability of atrial fibrillation (AF) recurrence.[76]

THE SOLUTION

Obstructive sleep apnea, an underdiagnosed condition characterized by intermittent pauses in breathing during sleep, affects about 15% of the US population.[77,78] Having obstructive sleep apnea nearly doubles the probability of AF recurrence after ablation; however, when treated with continuous positive airway pressure (CPAP), the risk that obstructive sleep apnea poses to AF recurrence is virtually eliminated.[76]

CPAP

A VICIOUS CYCLE

Obesity is a major risk factor for obstructive sleep apnea. Weight loss reduces sleep apnea symptom severity[79]; however, oxygen deprivation and sleep disruptions caused by sleep apnea exacerbate metabolic dysfunction, making it more difficult to lose weight, further highlighting the importance of CPAP.[78,80]

If you suspect you have sleep apnea, request a sleep study from your physician. Some smart devices can provide some information regarding sleep depth and blood oxygen levels during sleep; however, only a sleep study can lead to a diagnosis and treatment.

#9 SMOKING

SMOKING

CIGARETTE SMOKING

51% ↑RISK

***of* ATRIAL FIBRILLATION**[81]

The average smoking cessation success rate with a placebo or no drug is around 10.5%.[82-84]

Drug Therapy	Increase in Probability of Success*	Reference
Prescription-Only		
Bupropion	+8.0%	Howes et al.[83,85]
Nortriptyline	+10.1%	Hughes et al. [84,85]
Varenicline	+14.5%	Cahill et al. [85,86]
Nicotine Replacement Therapy		
Slow Acting		
Patch	+6.3%	Hartmann-Boyce et al. [82,85]
Fast Acting		
Gum	+6.3%	Hartmann-Boyce et al.[82,85]
Inhaler	+8.0%	Hartmann-Boyce et al.[82,85]
Tablets/Lozenges	+8.0%	Hartmann-Boyce et al.[82,85]
Nasal Spray	+12.1%	Hartmann-Boyce et al. [82,85]

*Increase in the absolute probability of success compared to placebo or no intervention.

Unless your physician says otherwise, smoking cessation medications should not be used in combination; however, there is an exception for nicotine replacement therapy (NRT). By combining one slow-acting NRT agent and one fast-acting NRT agent (e.g., patch (slow-acting) for basal nicotine and a fast-acting dosage form like the gum, inhaler, or nasal spray for immediate treatment of nicotine cravings), the probability of success increases by 3%.[87]

STRATEGIES TO BOOST THE PROBABILITY OF SUCCESS

Behavioral therapy (when added to drug therapy) may increase the probability of success by 2.4%.[82]
Support for medication adherence may increase the probability of success by 2.4%.[88]
Exercise may increase the probability of success by 1.3%.[89]

#10
MAGNESIUM

MAGNESIUM

"Magnesium therapy may be useful in the treatment of refractory ventricular tachycardia, ventricular fibrillation, multifocal atrial tachycardia, atrial fibrillation (AF), and supraventricular tachycardia."[90]

"The use of [magnesium] is promising... in preventing and treating cardiac arrhythmias, regulating blood pressure, and improving the function of the autonomic nervous system."[91]

RESEARCH FINDINGS

Individuals with relatively higher magnesium levels experience AF less frequently.[92]

A serum magnesium level ≥ 1.99 mg/dL was associated with a 33% lower risk of AF compared to those with a serum magnesium level ≤ 1.77 mg/dL.[93]

A serum magnesium level of 2.2 mg/dL has been associated with the lowest risk of AF.[92]

Note: Serum magnesium levels are constantly changing. Test results can vary from hour to hour.[94] The important point is that insufficient magnesium intake could increase the risk of AF.

ECTOPIC HEARTBEATS

Premature atrial contractions (or atrial "ectopic heartbeats") are associated with an increased risk of AF.[92] In a placebo-controlled trial, 77% of those taking a magnesium supplement had a >70% reduction in the number of ectopic heartbeats after 30 days of supplementation (compared to those taking a placebo).[95]

---

350 mg

MAXIMUM DAILY DOSE

The maximum daily dose of magnesium (from a supplement) is 350 milligrams.[96]

Note: Always check with your physician and pharmacist before taking a new supplement.

COMMON SIDE EFFECTS OF MAGNESIUM SUPPLEMENTS

✓ Diarrhea ✓ Nausea and vomiting ✓ Flatulence ✓ Dyspepsia

To minimize side effects, the daily dose of magnesium should be divided into smaller doses and taken with food multiple times a day (e.g., around 100 mg with a meal three times daily is appropriate in most situations). Note, however, that smaller doses, such as 100 mg once daily with breakfast, may also be useful to supplement a healthy diet.

WARNING: Individuals with impaired kidney function should not take magnesium supplements, as doing so could lead to hypermagnesemia, a potentially fatal condition. Always check with your physician and pharmacist before taking any supplements.

INFLAMMATION & BLOOD PRESSURE

The use of magnesium supplements is associated with significant reductions in various markers of inflammation[97] and blood pressure.[98]

MAGNESIUM ABSORPTION

A magnesium supplement must be taken by mouth and absorbed into the bloodstream to be beneficial. However, not all forms of magnesium are well-absorbed, and poorly absorbed forms can induce diarrhea and magnesium loss.[99] Therefore, the selection of the proper supplement is critical.

"Studies on the bioavailability of different magnesium salts consistently demonstrate that organic salts of magnesium have a higher bioavailability than inorganic salts..."[100]

GOOD ABSORPTION

ORGANIC
Magnesium citrate
Magnesium malate
Magnesium glycinate
Magnesium taurate
magnesium orotate

POOR ABSORPTION

INORGANIC
Magnesium oxide
Magnesium sulfate
Magnesium chloride
Magnesium carbonate

In one study evaluating the absorption of 15 magnesium supplements, the five supplements with the best absorption all contained an organic salt of magnesium. Meanwhile, the five supplements with the worst absorption all contained an inorganic salt of magnesium.[100] This further illustrates that organic salts of magnesium are absorbed to a greater extent. In this context, the term "organic" is a chemistry term that refers to compounds containing carbon-hydrogen or carbon-carbon bonds.

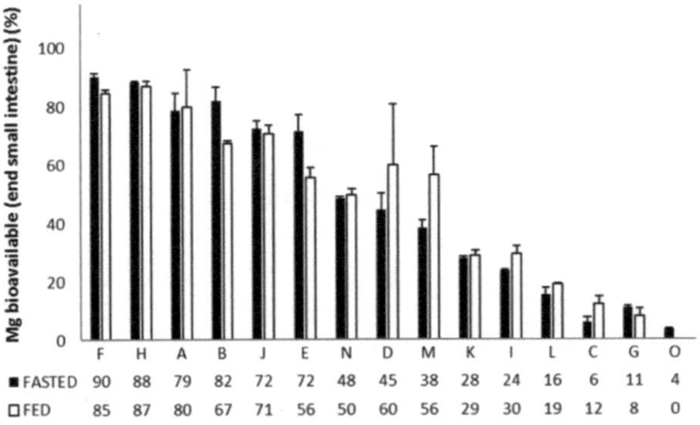

Code	Product	Manufacturer	Mg Content (mg)	Mg Salt	Pharmaceutical Form
A	Ultractive Magnesium	Oystershell	196	Mg oxide + Mg glycerophosphate	Tablet
B	MagnéVieB6	Sanofi-Aventis France	100	Mg citrate	Tablet
C	Promagnor	Merck	450	Mg oxide	Capsule
D	Mag 2	Cooper	100	Mg carbonate	Tablet
E	Magnesium Verla N tablets	Verla	40	Mg citrate + Mg bis (hydrogen-L-glutamate)	Tablet
F	Magnerot	Wörwag PHARMA	32.8	Mg orotate dihydrate	Tablet
G	Mag 2 24 h	Cooper	300	Mg oxide	Capsule
H	Polase	Pfizer	19	Mg citrate	Tablet
I	Biolectra	Hermes Arzneimittel	400	Mg oxide	Capsule
J	High Absorption Magnesium	Doctor's Best	100	Mg glycinate lysinate chelate	Tablet
K	MagOx 400	Akorn Consumer Health	241.3	Mg oxide	Tablet
L	Magnesium 500 mg	Nature's Bounty	500	Mg oxide	Tablet
M	Magnesium Citrate 200 mg	Now Foods	200	Mg citrate	Tablet
N	Slow-Mag	Purdue Products	71.5	Mg chloride	Tablet
O	B-Magnum	Merck	450	Mg oxide	Tablet

Graph and table from Blancquaert L, Vervaet C, Derave W. Predicting and Testing Bioavailability of Magnesium Supplements. Nutrients. 2019;11(7):1663. Published 2019 Jul 20. doi:10.3390/nu11071663, an open-access article distributed under the terms and conditions of the Creative Commons Attribution (CC BY) license.

HOW TO IDENTIFY HIGH-QUALITY SUPPLEMENTS

A study investigating the accuracy of supplement dosages demonstrated that in 58.7% of the magnesium supplements sampled, "the magnesium content was different than the permissible tolerance limits... It has been estimated that as a result of the differences in the content, the patient may take up to 304% more magnesium per day or 98% less than it is stated in the declaration."[101] In other words, the dose printed on the label of a magnesium supplement generally cannot be trusted as accurate. This illustrates just one of several commonly encountered issues with supplements.

Unlike the pharmaceutical industry, the dietary supplement industry is not tightly regulated. For this reason, pharmacists strongly recommend only using products that have been verified or certified by a reputable third-party organization. One example of such an organization is the United States Pharmacopeia (USP). USP operates a program that tests and audits dietary supplements for purity, potency, performance, and manufacturing practices. Supplements that pass all their tests can print the USP Verified Mark on their labels. NSF runs a similar program, and NSF-certified supplements display the NSF mark on their label.

The above symbols are registered trademarks of the respective organizations.
This book is neither affiliated with nor endorsed by these organizations.

A list of USP-verified supplements is available at: **quality-supplements.org/verified-products**
A list of NSF-certified supplements is available at: **info.nsf.org/Certified/dietary**

#11
POTASSIUM

POTASSIUM

Less than 2% of US adults consume the daily recommended amount of potassium (4,700 mg).[102,103]

The average daily potassium intake for an adult man is 3,016 mg, and for an adult woman is 2,320 mg.[104]

RESEARCH FINDINGS

Low serum potassium (< 3.5 mEq/L) is associated with a 63% higher incidence of AF compared to those with a normal serum potassium level (3.5-5.0 mEq/L).[105]

A large meta-analysis published in 2011 found that a 1,640-mg higher daily potassium intake was associated with a 21% lower risk of stroke.[106]

A NOTE ON THE INTERPRETATION OF POTASSIUM LAB RESULTS

Laboratories may express a serum potassium level in milliequivalents per liter (mEq/L) or millimoles per liter (mmol/L). In the case of potassium, no mathematical conversion is necessary (1 mEq/L = 1 mmol/L).

EXCELLENT SOURCES OF POTASSIUM

Whole foods (e.g., fresh fruits and vegetables) are the preferred source of potassium; however, other options include coconut water (approximately 575 mg/serving) and V8® Low Sodium Vegetable Juice (700 mg/serving).

POTASSIUM SUPPLEMENTS

Non-prescription potassium supplements should be avoided. The FDA limits the strength of potassium supplements to 99 mg of potassium per serving.[107] Furthermore, taking multiple servings is unsafe, as doing so can essentially burn a hole in the stomach lining. Alternatively, specially formulated prescription-only potassium supplements (e.g., Klor-Con®) provide relatively large doses of potassium; however, these are only appropriate for certain patients.

WARNING: In people with impaired kidney function or those taking medications that promote potassium retention, potassium intake should be increased cautiously and only after consulting a licensed physician.

THE CO-OPERATIONAL IMPORTANCE OF MAGNESIUM

Magnesium deficiency can drive potassium deficiency, as the kidneys utilize magnesium to regulate potassium levels.[103]

#12

COENZYME Q10

COENZYME Q10

Among other factors, oxidative stress and mitochondrial dysfunction have been implicated in the development and perpetuation of atrial fibrillation (AF).[108,109]

Coenzyme Q10 (CoQ10) possesses powerful antioxidant and anti-inflammatory properties.[110,111]

ANIMAL RESEARCH

Aldehyde dehydrogenase 2 (ALDH2) is a mitochondrial enzyme that is, among other functions, responsible for eliminating toxic chemicals generated from oxidative stress. About 8% of the world population produces a variant of ALDH2 known as ALDH2*2, which exhibits diminished catalytic activity and has been associated with cardiovascular disease. According to a 2021 study, "the treatment of ALDH2*2 mice with CoQ10 resulted in a 30% reduction in the incidence of AF... these results highlighted the suitability of CoQ10 to be used as a potential pharmacological agent to reduce the risk of AF."[112]

HUMAN RESEARCH

In a 2015 randomized controlled trial of 102 patients with heart failure, the use of CoQ10 30 mg per day for 12 months reduced the relative risk of experiencing AF by nearly 72%.[113]

A 2015 meta-analysis (involving just 70 patients) found that CoQ10 50-60 mg taken three times daily for 7-10 days before coronary artery bypass graft surgery reduced the incidence of ventricular arrhythmias by 95%.[114]

SAFETY CONSIDERATIONS

CoQ10 does not cause serious adverse effects and is considered "highly safe" as a dietary supplement at doses up to 1,200 mg/day.[115]

The chemical structure of CoQ10 resembles vitamin K and, therefore, may dangerously interact with Coumadin® (warfarin). Non-interacting alternatives to warfarin (e.g., Pradaxa®, Eliquis®, and Xarelto®) are available with a prescription. Always check with your physician and pharmacist before taking a supplement.

STANDARD VERSUS HIGH ABSORPTION FORMS OF CoQ10

Absorption issues are commonly cited by companies that sell high absorption CoQ10 formulations, probably in an attempt to gain a competitive advantage in the market (e.g., "our product is absorbed 100X better than regular CoQ10"). However, the above-cited research involved standard CoQ10. Therefore, standard CoQ10 should be preferred until further notice. In the meantime, purity and the general quality of the supplement are more important considerations. Pharmacists generally recommend supplements that are USP-verified or NSF certified.

BLOOD PRESSURE-LOWERING EFFECT

Beyond the potential arrhythmia-preventing effects, CoQ10 supplementation (at least 100 mg daily) has been shown to reduce systolic blood pressure by an average of 3.7 mmHg in individuals with hypertension.[116]

#13
QUERCETIN

QUERCETIN

Quercetin is a flavonoid polyphenol found in low concentrations in fruits and vegetables.[148] The average person in the United States consumes an estimated 25 mg of quercetin daily from food sources.[149] Quercetin intake can be boosted significantly through supplementation. The reasons to consider quercetin supplementation for atrial fibrillation (AF) prevention are illustrated by these quotes from three pertinent research papers:

> "Quercetin may alleviate AF by inhibiting fibrosis of atrial tissues..."[150]
>
> "In vivo results showed that quercetin significantly reduced the duration of AF and improved atrial remodeling, reduced p-MAPK protein expression, and inhibited the progression of AF."[151]
>
> "Quercetin can... significantly inhibit myocardial fibrosis and improve myocardial remodeling in AF."[152]

Quercetin has also been shown to decrease blood pressure and blood glucose while exhibiting antioxidant, antiviral, anti-microbial, anti-cancer, anti-inflammatory, cardioprotective, and neuroprotective effects."[153,154] Quercetin may also improve dental health, which may be important given the association between dental hygiene and AF.[149]

The use of quercetin does have drawbacks. For instance, quercetin supplementation may lower HDL cholesterol and raise triglycerides. As previously outlined, low HDL cholesterol and high triglycerides are both risk factors for AF. In one study, quercetin 150 mg taken daily for six weeks was associated with a 5.2% decrease in HDL and a 6.6% increase in triglycerides.[155]

SAFETY CONSIDERATIONS

Among the published human studies, side effects associated with quercetin have been rare and mild.[148]

"In human intervention studies, pro-oxidative effects of quercetin were not found with quercetin doses at 500–1,000 mg/day applied for 3–12 weeks, but it is still an open question whether quercetin may exhibit pro-oxidative effects in the human body, especially after a long-term use of high quercetin doses."[148]

In animal studies, high-dose quercetin has been associated with kidney damage and estrogen-dependent cancer.[148] Nonetheless, quercetin is not classified by the World Health Organization as a human carcinogen, and quercetin supplements continue to be commercially available in the US.[156]

In 2010, the US Food and Drug Administration (FDA) added quercetin 500 mg to a list of supplemental food/beverage ingredients generally recognized as safe.[157] However, quercetin is categorized as a dietary supplement, not a drug; therefore, under the Dietary Supplement Health and Education Act of 1994 (DSHEA), quercetin is categorized under the general umbrella of "foods."[158] According to the FDA website, some consequences of this categorization are as follows[158]:

1. "FDA does not have the authority to approve dietary supplements before they are marketed.
2. "Generally, a firm does not have to provide FDA with the evidence it relies on to substantiate safety before or after it markets its products..."
3. "FDA generally does not approve dietary supplement claims or other labeling before use."
4. "FDA has limited resources to analyze the composition of food products, including dietary supplements, and, therefore, focuses its resources first on public health emergencies and products that may have caused injury or illness."

Unlike coenzyme Q10, which has some limited clinical research to support its use, we still don't have clinical trials on quercetin for AF. Therefore, at the time of this writing, quercetin is perhaps the most speculative intervention outlined in this book.

#14
GREEN TEA

GREEN TEA

Researchers have hypothesized that a prominent flavonoid in green tea, epigallocatechin gallate (EGCG), may protect the heart against oxidation and fibrosis.[117]

HUMAN RESEARCH

In a Chinese study of 801 subjects, green tea consumption was associated with a 65% lower incidence of AF.[117] Those who consumed "low-dose" green tea benefited the most.

The term "low-dose" was defined by three factors:

1. Low frequency (less than one cup a day)
2. Low concentration (tea leaves < 25% of the volume of the cup)
3. Low duration (1–15 years).

The apparent protective effect weakened as green tea consumption increased. The authors of this study speculate that the large amounts of caffeine consumed from higher doses of green tea may counter the beneficial effects of EGCG, thus accounting for the reduced benefit at higher doses.[117]

ANIMAL RESEARCH

The idea that EGCG could protect against AF is supported by a 2015 animal study in which rabbits treated with EGCG were found to have lower levels of inflammation, oxidative stress, and atrial fibrosis. The researchers found it more difficult to induce AF in the EGCG-treated rabbits, and when AF was induced, the episodes were shorter than those in the untreated rabbits.[118]

FRESH-BREWED vs. BOTTLED GREEN TEA

According to the Phenol-Explorer Database (http://phenol-explorer.eu), the concentration of EGCG in bottled green tea is less than one-third of that in freshly brewed green tea. Of all types of tea, fresh-brewed green tea contains the highest amount of EGCG and the lowest amount of caffeine.

BLOOD PRESSURE-LOWERING EFFECT

A meta-analysis of 25 randomized controlled trials concluded that green tea lowers blood pressure.[119]

ANTI-INFLAMMATORY EFFECT

Teas and herbal infusions ("herbal teas") possess anti-inflammatory properties.[42]

#15
DENTAL HYGEINE

DENTAL HYGIENE

"Poor dental health is associated with high levels of inflammation, poor diet quality, and conditions such as disability, diabetes, and increased risk of cardiovascular disease and pneumonia."[120]

CONSEQUENCES OF POOR DENTAL HYGIENE

"Poor oral hygiene can provoke transient bacteremia and systemic inflammation, a mediator of atrial fibrillation (AF) and heart failure."[121]

"Poor oral hygiene is... associated with continuous systemic inflammation leading to a raised concentration of CRP and other inflammatory biomarkers... An elevated CRP level was associated with a higher risk of the development of AF, increased AF burden, and higher recurrence rate after electrical cardioversion and radiofrequency catheter ablation."[122]

BRUSH TEETH

Compared to brushing less than twice a day, brushing twice a day was associated with a 5% lower risk of AF, and brushing ≥ 3 times/day was associated with a 10% lower risk of AF.[121]

According to a Delta Dental survey, 2% of the population does not brush at all, 27% brush once daily, 57% twice daily, and 14% three or more times daily.[123]

PROFESSIONAL DENTAL CLEANING

In a Taiwan study of several thousand people with no history of cardiac arrhythmias, those who received "dental scaling" (professional dental cleaning) at least once a year for three consecutive years were 32.9% less likely to be diagnosed with new-onset AF compared to those who received no dental scaling.[122]

The apparent AF-protective benefit was much stronger in those who received twice-yearly dental cleanings than those who received only one professional dental cleaning per year.[122]

ROUTINE FLOSSING & ELECTRIC TOOTHBRUSH

Although the relationship between flossing and AF has not been studied, it stands to reason that additional AF-protective effects might be derived from routine (e.g., nightly) flossing. Following the same logic, using an electric toothbrush could also reasonably be expected to provide an advantage.[124]

A DIET RICH IN POLYPHENOLS

"Consistent studies showing that polyphenols inactivate periodontal pathogens, and increase antioxidant capacity of oral fluids, suggest a preventive effect against periodontal disease with fair evidence."[125]
The Mediterranean diet is rich in polyphenols.[126]

#16
ACID REFLUX

ACID REFLUX

"The notion that atrial fibrillation (AF) and gastroesophageal reflux disease (GERD) are mutually interdependent is widely and empirically recognized."[127]

The heart is located near the stomach and esophagus. Consequently, issues such as GERD and hiatal hernia may physically or biochemically affect the heart, triggering or otherwise promoting AF.[128]

According to a 2019 meta-analysis, GERD may increase the risk of AF by 6%.[129] While the mechanism linking GERD to AF is unclear, measures to avoid or mitigate acid reflux represent another possible opportunity to reduce AF risk.

ACID-REDUCING MEDICATIONS

Proton pump inhibitors (e.g., Prilosec® (omeprazole) and Protonix® (pantoprazole)) represent the most effective class of acid suppressants, reducing gastric acid production by 80-95%.[130] Next most effective is the H2 blockers (e.g., Pepcid® (famotidine), reducing gastric acid production by around 70%. Unfortunately, both classes of medication have been associated with magnesium depletion.[131,132] As highlighted in this book, low serum magnesium may increase AF risk. While using these medications short-term (or long-term if under medical supervision) may be necessary and appropriate, effective non-drug alternatives exist.

COMMON NON-DRUG STRATEGIES FOR PREVENTING GERD

Reduce abdominal mass (i.e., lose excess weight), avoid foods and beverages that trigger acid reflux, elevate the head of the bed or use a wedge pillow, and stop smoking (if applicable).[133]

DO NOT EAT BEFORE GOING TO BED

Eat dinner four or more hours before bedtime, and do not eat again after dinner. Eating dinner within three hours of bedtime (as opposed to four or more hours) was associated with a more than 7X higher risk of GERD.[134]

THE MEDITERRANEAN DIET

One study demonstrated that a non-Mediterranean diet was associated with a 2.3X higher risk of GERD.[135]

Another study compared a proton pump inhibitor to a combination of alkaline water and a 90% plant-based Mediterranean-style diet. The group that received the proton pump inhibitor recorded a 27.2% reduction in the reflux symptom index; meanwhile, the group treated with alkaline water (pH > 8) and a 90% plant-based Mediterranean-style diet recorded a 39.8% reduction in the reflux symptom index.[136] Note that, in addition to their respective treatments, everyone in the study also followed "standard reflux precautions," which included abstaining from coffee, tea, chocolate, soda, alcohol, and greasy, fried, fatty, and spicy foods.[136]

#17
ANTIOXIDANTS

DIETARY ANTIOXIDANTS

"It is widely accepted that a plant-based diet with high intake of fruits, vegetables, and other nutrient-rich plant foods may reduce the risk of oxidative stress-related diseases."[137]

TOP 10 SOURCES OF ANTIOXIDANTS IN THE AVERAGE US DIET[138]

Food/beverage	Antioxidant consumption per day[138]
Coffee	1,299 mg
Black tea	294 mg
Bananas	76 mg
Dry beans	72 mg
Corn	48 mg
Red wine	44 mg
Lager beer	42 mg
Apples	39 mg
Tomatoes	32 mg
Potatoes	28 mg
Total	1,974 mg

*The antioxidant values from this source appear to be based on average consumption in the United States (US). For instance, the average person in the US consumes 65 apples per year, equivalent to 0.178 apples per day. The antioxidant content of one apple is estimated to be 221 mg; therefore, the average person consumes 39 mg of antioxidants from apples each day on average (221 mg/apple x 0.178 apples/day = 39 mg).

THE STANDARD AMERICAN DIET

"The Standard American Diet (SAD) has long been implicated in contributing to the health challenges experienced in the United States. Significant changes to the SAD have occurred since the 1950s, including a greater abundance and accessibility to calorie-dense and nutrient-poor food and beverage choices."[139]

"The poor diets and sedentary lifestyles of the American public have led to high rates of obesity, overweight, and diet-related chronic diseases..."[140]

Darker-pigmented plant foods tend to contain more antioxidants.[141]
Select examples are outlined below.

White onions → 13 mg of antioxidants/serving
Yellow onions → 23 mg of antioxidants/serving
Red onions → 31 mg of antioxidants/serving

Green grapes → 66 mg of antioxidants/serving
Black grapes → 92 mg of antioxidants/serving

White beans → 121 mg of antioxidants/serving
Black beans → 1,216 mg of antioxidants/serving

Green lettuce → 16 mg of antioxidants/serving
Red lettuce → 27 mg of antioxidants/serving

The next page lists some of the richest dietary sources of antioxidants.

DIETARY ANTIOXIDANTS

	Item	Antioxidant content[141]
FRUITS	Blackberries	821 mg/serving
	Wild blueberries	678 mg/serving
	Strawberries	480 mg/serving
	Plums	349 mg/serving
	Blueberries	321 mg/serving
	Sweet cherries	249 mg/serving
	Apples	221 mg/serving
	Red raspberries	213 mg/serving
	Bananas	150 mg/serving
	Pears	149 mg/serving
BEVERAGES	Coffee (filtered)	507 mg/serving
	Pure pomegranate juice	306 mg/serving
	Black tea	204 mg/serving
	Green tea	121 mg/serving
NUT & SEEDS	Chestnuts	524 mg/serving
	Walnuts	473 mg/serving
	Flaxseed (ground/milled)	306 mg/serving
	Pecans	272 mg/serving
	Hazelnut	192 mg/serving
BEANS	Black beans	1,216 mg/serving
	White beans	121 mg/serving
VEGETABLES	Globe artichoke heads	1,918 mg/serving
	Spinach	170 mg/serving
	Broccoli	142 mg/serving
	Green beans	185mg/serving
COCOA	Dark chocolate	316 mg/serving
	Cocoa powder	55 mg/serving
SPICES & HERBS	Cloves	802 mg/5 grams
	Ceylon cinnamon	454 mg/5 grams
	Spearmint (dried)	329 mg/5 grams
	Sweet basil (dried)	216 mg/5 grams
	Marjoram (dried)	192 mg/5 grams
	Sage (dried)	146 mg/5 grams
	Rosemary (dried)	126 mg/5 grams
	Cumin	102 mg/5 grams
	Thyme (dried)	91 mg/5 grams
	Parsley (dried)	79 mg /5 grams
	Curry powder	54 mg/5 grams
	Peppermint (dried)	49 mg/5 grams
	Ginger (dried)	24 mg/5 grams

Note: Cassia cinnamon, the type most often sold in the United States, contains a higher concentration of coumarins which, if consumed in large amounts, can increase the risk of bleeding. Additionally, foods and beverages rich in vitamin K (e.g., spinach, broccoli, green tea) can interfere with the effect of warfarin. Therefore, if taking warfarin, consult your healthcare provider before increasing the consumption of these items.

AMLA

In an analysis of the antioxidant content of 3,139 foods, beverages, spices, herbs, and supplements, AMLA (Indian gooseberry) was the second richest source of antioxidants, with over 100X more antioxidants than filtered coffee.[137] AMLA is both bitter and sour; however, only a small amount (2-3 grams/day) could impart significant health benefits. Furthermore, the taste of AMLA can be masked by mixing it with other food or blending it in a smoothie. Of interest to those attempting to minimize their risk of AF, just 2-3 grams of AMLA powder (dried Indian gooseberry) taken once daily after breakfast had the following effects[142]:

1. Up to 44% increase in HDL cholesterol
2. Up to 36% reduction in triglycerides
3. Up to 28% reduction in blood glucose 2 hours after a meal

Note: The above-outlined changes were even more significant in patients with diabetes.

AMLA also appears to have anti-cancer, anti-inflammatory, and neuroprotective properties.[143]

ANTIOXIDANT SUPPLEMENTS

LONG-TERM ANTIOXIDANT SUPPLEMENTATION

"The majority of [antioxidant] supplementation studies indicate no variation of general mortality and of cancer incidence or a detrimental effect on both. Antioxidant supplements so far tested seem to offer no improvement over a well-balanced diet..."[144]

SHORT-TERM ANTIOXIDANT SUPPLEMENTATION

In a meta-analysis of eight randomized controlled trials (including 1,060 participants), the risk of postoperative AF was 53% lower in the group that received vitamin C (compared to placebo).[145] This meta-analysis, however, did not include two of the largest trials on vitamin C supplementation and AF, both of which found no effect.[146] These larger trials with null findings were not included in the meta-analysis because they were never published. This is an excellent example of how publication bias can skew our perception of reality (see page 8). Yet, years after the problems with this meta-analysis were formally identified, the original paper still has not been retracted by the publisher, and it probably never will be.

COFFEE

5+ CUPS of COFFEE/DAY
10% ↓RISK *of* ATRIAL FIBRILLATION

A 2021 meta-analysis of 12 observational cohort studies found no statistically significant correlation between coffee or caffeine intake and AF risk. However, when studies with a moderate risk of bias were excluded from the analysis, it was determined that those who consumed five or more cups of coffee per day were 10% less likely to develop new-onset AF than those who consumed just one to two cups of coffee per day.[147] As mentioned in the "AF Triggers" section, many have reported coffee as an AF trigger. So, as with all the interventions outlined in this book, the decision of whether to consume coffee for its potential AF-preventive properties should be made on an individual basis.

#18
PREBIOTICS & PROBIOTICS

PREBIOTICS & PROBIOTICS

Prebiotics are components of food that promote the growth of beneficial gut bacteria, such as the fructans found in bananas, tomatoes, and onions.[7]

Probiotics, on the other hand, are live bacteria introduced into the gastrointestinal tract (e.g., fermented foods/beverages) by ingestion.[7]

Atrial fibrillation (AF) is associated with a disordered gut microbiota. "Preventative and therapeutic measures targeting gut microbiota for early intervention to postpone the progression of AF are highly warranted."[159]

"Most studies have only found an association between gut microbiota disturbances and AF, but the causal relationship requires further verification."[160] While more research is needed to determine what role probiotics may play in preventing or treating AF, research has already demonstrated that probiotic supplementation reduces blood sugar, lowers blood pressure, and possibly raises HDL cholesterol levels in some patients.[161] High blood sugar, high blood pressure, and low HDL cholesterol are all risk factors for AF.

The human gut is host to around 300-500 species of bacteria that collectively outnumber all other cells in the human body by about 10X.[162] As one might imagine, the subject of gut microbiota is tremendously complex.

Rather than purchase an expensive probiotic supplement that may or may not deliver a benefit, consider consuming probiotic and prebiotic foods and beverages.

SELECT EXAMPLES OF PREBIOTIC FOODS

Fruits, vegetables, asparagus, sugar beet, garlic, chicory, onion, Jerusalem artichoke, wheat, banana, barley, tomato, rye, blue agave, leeks, bamboo shoots, honey, wheat bran, and cocoa.[7,163]

Note: "...although not all dietary fibers are prebiotics, all prebiotics are dietary fibers."[164]

SELECT EXAMPLES OF PROBIOTIC FOODS AND BEVERAGES

Fermented dairy products (yogurt, cheese, kefir), fermented tea (kombucha), fermented cabbage (sauerkraut, kimchi), fermented soybean products (tempeh, miso, and natto), and sourdough bread.[165]

#19

POLLUTION

AIR POLLUTION

Air pollution may increase the risk of developing AF; however, research has produced mixed results, so what can be said at this point is that air pollution either increases the risk of AF or doesn't. In any case, it does not reduce the risk. For that reason, it's reasonable to take measures to avoid exposure, particularly long-term exposure.

In one study, researchers found that a 3.9-µg/m³ increase in the 3-year average $PM_{2.5}$ (fine inhalable particles with a diameter of 2.5 micrometers or less) was associated with an 8% increased risk of AF.[166] Another study showed an 18% increase in AF for each 10-µg/m³ increase in $PM_{2.5}$.[167] However, only mentioning these studies would be cherry-picking. Other research has found no association between air pollution and AF risk.

Firefighters are exposed to heavily polluted air each time they fight fires (e.g., smoke, volatile organic compounds). In a survey of 10,860 firefighters, those who fought 31 or more fires per year were more than twice as likely to report AF than those who fought five or fewer.[168]

BreezoMeter (breezometer.com/air-quality-map) can provide a comprehensive analysis of the current air quality in your area. Consider using an air purifier that can filter out fine particulate matter, including $PM_{2.5}$, especially if you live in an area where air pollution is problematic.

NOISE POLLUTION

Additional research is needed to determine whether environmental noise impacts the likelihood of developing AF. However, in a study of 23,528 Danish nurses, living in an area where the average road traffic noise level was > 58 decibels (dB) was associated with an 18% higher risk of developing AF (compared to those living in an area where the noise level was < 48 dB).[166] In another published study of the same group, a 25-30% higher risk of AF was seen in those exposed to long-term wind turbine noise of 20 dB or higher. While the association was seen with noise exposure during the day and night, nighttime noise exposure had a slightly stronger association with the development of AF.[169]

National Institute for Occupational Safety & Health (NIOSH) offers a free sound level meter smartphone app for Apple devices. A similar app is available for Android devices.

#20
OCCUPATION

JOB STRAIN

High-strain jobs (i.e., "exposure to occupational psychosocial stress") were associated with a 23% higher risk of developing atrial fibrillation (AF).[170] To determine job strain, researchers used the Swedish job exposure matrix published in the late 1970s, which analyzed 261 jobs and provided estimates of demand and control. High-strain jobs were characterized by a high level of demand and a low level of control.

DEMAND

Question #1 Is your job hectic? Question #2 Is your job psychologically demanding?
If you answered "yes" to both questions, your occupation is "high demand."
If you answered "yes" to one question, your occupation is "moderate demand."
If you answered "no" to both questions, your occupation is "low demand."

CONTROL

Control is determined by a combination of factors, such as intellectual discretion and personal schedule freedom (e.g., the freedom to complete personal tasks while at work). "High-control" occupations are considered less stressful than "low-control" occupations.

According to the demand-control model, there are four job categories.[171]

1. Low strain (low demand, high control)
2. Passive (low demand, low control)
3. Active (high demand, high control)
4. High strain (high demand, low control)

Occupational psychosocial stress can also be estimated, perhaps capturing more nuance than the demand-control model, using data from O*NET (onetonline.org), a free online database of more than 1,000 occupations.

For example, to rank occupations by various criteria related to stress, do the following:
Go to onetonline.org > O*NET Data > Work Styles > Expand All > Stress Tolerance
Go to onetonline.org > O*NET Data > Work Context > Expand All > Frequency of Conflict Situations
Go to onetonline.org > O*NET Data > Work Context > Expand All > Deal with Unpleasant or Angry People
Go to onetonline.org > O*NET Data > Work Context > Expand All > Deal with Physically Aggressive People
Go to onetonline.org > O*NET Data > Work Context > Expand All > Time Pressure

---

#21
PSYCHOLOGY

PSYCHOLOGY

ANGER, HOSTILITY, AND TENSION

Symptoms of anger were associated with a 20% increase in the risk of developing AF.[172]
Hostility was associated with a 30% increase in the risk of developing AF.[172]
Tension was associated with a 24% increase in the risk of developing AF.[173]
Note: These associations were observed in men but not women.

PSYCHOLOGICAL STATES ASSOCIATED WITH AF EPISODE ONSET[174]		
Lower Risk of AF Episode	Happiness	88% lower risk of AF episode onset
	Hunger	2% lower risk of AF episode onset
Higher Risk of AF Episode	Sadness	5X higher risk of AF episode onset
	Anger	4X higher risk of AF episode onset
	Stress	3X higher risk of AF episode onset
	Impatience	3X higher risk of AF episode onset
	Anxiety	4X higher risk of AF episode onset

A VICIOUS CYCLE

AF can cause anxiety and depression. Meanwhile, anxiety and depression appear to increase the likelihood of AF episodes. It's a vicious cycle.

THE PSYCHOLOGICAL IMPACT OF ATRIAL FIBRILLATION

Among 78 patients with AF, 35% reported severe anxiety and distress, and 20% reported suicidal thoughts.[19]

"This psychological impact [of AF] is not well appreciated by many heart specialists..."[19]
-Professor Jonathan M. Kalman, MBBS, PhD

THE IMPORTANCE OF A HEALTHY DIETARY PATTERN

In the first study examining the potential association between pro-inflammatory food consumption and the risk of psychological disorders, women with a dietary pattern representative of the top 20% of the food-based dietary inflammatory index (FDII) had a 49% higher risk of depression, 92% higher risk of anxiety, and 68% higher risk of psychological distress (compared to women with a dietary pattern representative of the bottom 20% of the FDII). However, the study found no association between FDII and psychological disorders in men.[175]

#22
YOGA

YOGA

In a clinical trial with 49 symptomatic paroxysmal atrial fibrillation (AF) patients, each underwent an initial three-month observation period followed by three months of twice-weekly 60-minute yoga training sessions. Data was collected during the initial three-month observation period, allowing each participant to serve as their own control.[16]

THE EFFECT *of* YOGA ON AF[16]

↓23.7%	↓33.3%
symptomatic AF episodes	symptomatic non-AF episodes

"Symptomatic non-AF episodes" were those in which the participants experienced symptoms of AF, but electrocardiogram (ECG) recordings revealed that they, in fact, were not in AF.

YOGA TRAINING PROGRAM FEATURES[16]

Participants met in a yoga studio in groups of 15-20 with 60-minute training sessions led by a certified professional yoga instructor. The sessions were structured as follows:

Pranayamas (10 minutes)
Warm-up exercises (10 minutes)
Asanas (30 minutes)
Relaxation exercises (10 minutes)

Twenty-two percent (22%) of participants, each with an active AF diagnosis, experienced zero documented episodes of AF during the 3-month yoga phase of the trial.[16]

THE HEALTH BENEFITS OF YOGA

PSYCHOLOGICAL BENEFITS[16]	CARDIOVASCULAR BENEFITS[16]	GENERAL HEALTH BENEFITS[16]
Depression scores ↓6.9%	Heart rate ↓4.9%	Physical functioning ↑5.9%
Anxiety scores ↓24.2%	Systolic blood pressure ↓4%	General health ↑25%
Mental health ↑6.7%	Diastolic blood pressure ↓5.4%	Vitality ↑8.3%
	↑ High blood pressure is the single most impactful risk factor leading to the development of AF.[6]	

#23
SLEEP

SLEEP PATTERN

In a study of more than 400,000 participants, healthier sleep patterns were associated with a lower risk of developing AF.[176]

The five components of a healthy sleep pattern[176]:

1. Never, rarely, or only sometimes unintentionally falling asleep during the day
2. Never or rarely experience trouble falling or staying asleep
3. Sleeping 7-8 hours per day (including naps)
4. Possessing an early chronotype (i.e., more of a morning person than an evening person)
5. Not snoring (according to partner, close relative, or friend)

DETERMINE YOUR SLEEP PATTERN[176]
Step 1: Select one response from each of the five areas.

How often do you unintentionally fall asleep during the day?

Never/rarely (1 point)	Sometimes (1 point)	Often (0 points)	All the time (0 points)

How often do you have trouble falling asleep or staying asleep at night?

Never (1 point)	Rarely (1 point)	Sometimes (1 point)	Usually (0 points)

How many hours of sleep (including naps) do you normally get per day?

<7 hours per day (0 points)	7-8 hours per day (1 point)	>8 hours per day (0 points)

Are you more of a morning person or an evening person?

Morning person (1 point)	Evening person (0 points)

Do you snore according to your partner, close relative, or friend?

No (1 point)	Yes (0 points)

Step 2: Add up your points.
A score of 0 or 1 point was used as the reference point.
A score of 2 points was associated with a 14% lower risk of developing AF.
A score of 3 points was associated with a 21% lower risk of developing AF.
A score of 4 points was associated with a 28% lower risk of developing AF.
A score of 5 points was associated with a 29% lower risk of developing AF.

NIGHT SHIFT WORK

A study observing more than 280,000 participants found that, compared to working only during the day, those who worked a lifetime average of 3-8 night shifts per month were 22% more likely to develop AF and 35% more likely to develop coronary heart disease.[177]

MISCELLANEOUS

ATRIAL FIBRILLATION TRIGGERS

According to responses from a survey of one hundred people with paroxysmal atrial fibrillation (AF), the factors that most commonly triggered AF were[178]: #1 Mental stress, #2 Physical exertion, #3 Fatigue, #4 Alcohol, #5 Coffee, and #6 Infection.

STRATEGIES FOR REDUCING EXPOSURE TO AF TRIGGERS

1) minimize and combat mental stress 2) gradually achieve and maintain physical fitness 3) develop a healthy sleeping pattern 4) abstain from alcohol 5) consider decaffeinated coffee (only if coffee is a trigger, as some research suggests regular coffee may have a protective effect) 6) wash hands frequently, maintain good personal hygiene, and take reasonable measures to avoid infection.

THE KEY TO LONG-TERM ABLATION SUCCESS

What is the key to long-term ablation success? Is it information? No! In the LEGACY and ARREST-AF trials, more than 80% of the groups that received information only (the control groups) experienced AF recurrence. Information was not the differentiator. The differentiator was participation in a risk factor management program.

A NOTE TO THOSE WITH "BAD GENETICS"

A subset of the population will develop AF despite having no apparent risk factors. The term "lone atrial fibrillation" (or "lone AF") has been used to describe AF in these individuals, particularly those who are young. Several studies indicate that lone AF may be a consequence of genetics.[179] What if you spend a great deal of time and effort optimizing your modifiable AF risk factors, only to develop AF anyway? Obviously, that would be frustrating and demoralizing; however, aggressively targeting modifiable AF risk factors has the broader effect of improving your overall health. The better your overall health, the less likely you are to experience serious complications from AF, life-threatening complications from cardiac catheter ablation, and AF recurrence after a successful ablation.

If genetics heighten your risk of developing AF, are you truly doomed? Consider this. In people with a genetic profile that placed them at high risk for cardiovascular events, a favorable lifestyle reduced their risk of coronary events by nearly 50%.[180] A "favorable lifestyle" in this study was defined by four factors: #1 no current smoking, #2 BMI < 30 kg/m^2, #3 physical activity at least once weekly, and #4 a healthy dietary pattern. It is conceivable that a more aggressively managed lifestyle might have produced even better results.

THE END

CITATIONS

1. Xiong XJ, Wang PQ, Li SJ, Li XK, Zhang YQ, Wang J. Garlic for hypertension: A systematic review and meta-analysis of randomized controlled trials. *Phytomedicine*. Mar 15 2015;22(3):352-61. doi:10.1016/j.phymed.2014.12.013
2. Aune D, Feng T, Schlesinger S, Janszky I, Norat T, Riboli E. Diabetes mellitus, blood glucose and the risk of atrial fibrillation: A systematic review and meta-analysis of cohort studies. *J Diabetes Complications*. 05 2018;32(5):501-511. doi:10.1016/j.jdiacomp.2018.02.004
3. Alonso A, Yin X, Roetker NS, et al. Blood lipids and the incidence of atrial fibrillation: the Multi-Ethnic Study of Atherosclerosis and the Framingham Heart Study. *J Am Heart Assoc*. Oct 07 2014;3(5):e001211. doi:10.1161/JAHA.114.001211
4. Pathak RK, Middeldorp ME, Meredith M, et al. Long-Term Effect of Goal-Directed Weight Management in an Atrial Fibrillation Cohort: A Long-Term Follow-Up Study (LEGACY). *J Am Coll Cardiol*. May 26 2015;65(20):2159-69. doi:10.1016/j.jacc.2015.03.002
5. Donnellan E, Wazni OM, Harb S, Kanj M, Saliba WI, Jaber WA. Higher baseline cardiorespiratory fitness is associated with lower arrhythmia recurrence and death after atrial fibrillation ablation. *Heart Rhythm*. 10 2020;17(10):1687-1693. doi:10.1016/j.hrthm.2020.05.013
6. Verdecchia P, Angeli F, Reboldi G. Hypertension and Atrial Fibrillation: Doubts and Certainties From Basic and Clinical Studies. *Circ Res*. Jan 19 2018;122(2):352-368. doi:10.1161/CIRCRESAHA.117.311402
7. Green M, Arora K, Prakash S. Microbial Medicine: Prebiotic and Probiotic Functional Foods to Target Obesity and Metabolic Syndrome. *Int J Mol Sci*. Apr 21 2020;21(8)doi:10.3390/ijms21082890
8. O'Keefe EL, Sturgess JE, O'Keefe JH, Gupta S, Lavie CJ. Prevention and Treatment of Atrial Fibrillation via Risk Factor Modification. *Am J Cardiol*. 12 01 2021;160:46-52. doi:10.1016/j.amjcard.2021.08.042
9. Kunutsor SK, Seidu S, Mäkikallio TH, Dey RS, Laukkanen JA. Physical activity and risk of atrial fibrillation in the general population: meta-analysis of 23 cohort studies involving about 2 million participants. *Eur J Epidemiol*. Mar 2021;36(3):259-274. doi:10.1007/s10654-020-00714-4
10. Virani SS, Alonso A, Benjamin EJ, et al. Heart Disease and Stroke Statistics-2020 Update: A Report From the American Heart Association. *Circulation*. 03 03 2020;141(9):e139-e596. doi:10.1161/CIR.0000000000000757
11. Heron M. Deaths: Leading Causes for 2017. *Natl Vital Stat Rep*. Jun 2019;68(6):1-77.
12. Fauchier L, Villejoubert O, Clementy N, et al. Causes of Death and Influencing Factors in Patients with Atrial Fibrillation. *Am J Med*. Dec 2016;129(12):1278-1287. doi:10.1016/j.amjmed.2016.06.045
13. Reiffel JA. Atrial fibrillation and stroke: epidemiology. *Am J Med*. Apr 2014;127(4):e15-6. doi:10.1016/j.amjmed.2013.06.002
14. Du X, Dong J, Ma C. Is Atrial Fibrillation a Preventable Disease? *J Am Coll Cardiol*. Apr 18 2017;69(15):1968-1982. doi:10.1016/j.jacc.2017.02.020
15. McKay DL, Chen CY, Saltzman E, Blumberg JB. Hibiscus sabdariffa L. tea (tisane) lowers blood pressure in prehypertensive and mildly hypertensive adults. *J Nutr*. Feb 2010;140(2):298-303. doi:10.3945/jn.109.115097
16. Lakkireddy D, Atkins D, Pillarisetti J, et al. Effect of yoga on arrhythmia burden, anxiety, depression, and quality of life in paroxysmal atrial fibrillation: the YOGA My Heart Study. *J Am Coll Cardiol*. Mar 19 2013;61(11):1177-82. doi:10.1016/j.jacc.2012.11.060
17. Appel LJ, Moore TJ, Obarzanek E, et al. A clinical trial of the effects of dietary patterns on blood pressure. DASH Collaborative Research Group. *N Engl J Med*. Apr 17 1997;336(16):1117-24. doi:10.1056/NEJM199704173361601
18. Buckley BJR, Lip GYH, Thijssen DHJ. The counterintuitive role of exercise in the prevention and cause of atrial fibrillation. *Am J Physiol Heart Circ Physiol*. 11 01 2020;319(5):H1051-H1058. doi:10.1152/ajpheart.00509.2020
19. News AHA. Common treatment for AFib may lower anxiety, depression. American Heart Association. Accessed August 28, 2022, 2022. https://www.heart.org/en/news/2018/09/18/common-treatment-for-afib-may-lower-anxiety-depression
20. Pathak RK, Middeldorp ME, Lau DH, et al. Aggressive risk factor reduction study for atrial fibrillation and implications for the outcome of ablation: the ARREST-AF cohort study. *J Am Coll Cardiol*. Dec 02 2014;64(21):2222-31. doi:10.1016/j.jacc.2014.09.028

21. Chung MK, Eckhardt LL, Chen LY, et al. Lifestyle and Risk Factor Modification for Reduction of Atrial Fibrillation: A Scientific Statement From the American Heart Association. *Circulation*. 04 21 2020;141(16):e750-e772. doi:10.1161/CIR.0000000000000748
22. Tenny S, Varacallo M. StatPearls. 2023.
23. Guyatt GH, Sackett DL, Sinclair JC, Hayward R, Cook DJ, Cook RJ. Users' guides to the medical literature. IX. A method for grading health care recommendations. Evidence-Based Medicine Working Group. *JAMA*. Dec 13 1995;274(22):1800-4. doi:10.1001/jama.274.22.1800
24. Carlisle JB. False individual patient data and zombie randomised controlled trials submitted to Anaesthesia. *Anaesthesia*. Apr 2021;76(4):472-479. doi:10.1111/anae.15263
25. Lose G, Klarskov N. Why published research is untrustworthy. *Int Urogynecol J*. Sep 2017;28(9):1271-1274. doi:10.1007/s00192-017-3389-1
26. Hopewell S, Loudon K, Clarke MJ, Oxman AD, Dickersin K. Publication bias in clinical trials due to statistical significance or direction of trial results. *Cochrane Database Syst Rev*. Jan 21 2009;2009(1):MR000006. doi:10.1002/14651858.MR000006.pub3
27. Cook DJ, Guyatt GH, Ryan G, et al. Should unpublished data be included in meta-analyses? Current convictions and controversies. *JAMA*. Jun 02 1993;269(21):2749-53.
28. on NAUCoMEaOR, Investments FR. Measuring the Impacts of Federal Investments in Research: A Workshop Summary. 2011.
29. Bhandari M, Busse JW, Jackowski D, et al. Association between industry funding and statistically significant pro-industry findings in medical and surgical randomized trials. *CMAJ*. Feb 17 2004;170(4):477-80.
30. Larsson SC, Drca N, Jensen-Urstad M, Wolk A. Chocolate consumption and risk of atrial fibrillation: Two cohort studies and a meta-analysis. *Am Heart J*. Jan 2018;195:86-90. doi:10.1016/j.ahj.2017.09.013
31. Nicholls SJ, Lincoff AM, Garcia M, et al. Effect of High-Dose Omega-3 Fatty Acids vs Corn Oil on Major Adverse Cardiovascular Events in Patients at High Cardiovascular Risk: The STRENGTH Randomized Clinical Trial. *JAMA*. Dec 08 2020;324(22):2268-2280. doi:10.1001/jama.2020.22258
32. Albert CM, Cook NR, Pester J, et al. Effect of Marine Omega-3 Fatty Acid and Vitamin D Supplementation on Incident Atrial Fibrillation: A Randomized Clinical Trial. *JAMA*. 03 16 2021;325(11):1061-1073. doi:10.1001/jama.2021.1489
33. Pathak RK, Elliott A, Middeldorp ME, et al. Impact of CARDIOrespiratory FITness on Arrhythmia Recurrence in Obese Individuals With Atrial Fibrillation: The CARDIO-FIT Study. *J Am Coll Cardiol*. Sep 01 2015;66(9):985-96. doi:10.1016/j.jacc.2015.06.488
34. Wong CX, Sullivan T, Sun MT, et al. Obesity and the Risk of Incident, Post-Operative, and Post-Ablation Atrial Fibrillation: A Meta-Analysis of 626,603 Individuals in 51 Studies. *JACC Clin Electrophysiol*. Jun 2015;1(3):139-152. doi:10.1016/j.jacep.2015.04.004
35. Dublin S, French B, Glazer NL, et al. Risk of new-onset atrial fibrillation in relation to body mass index. *Arch Intern Med*. Nov 27 2006;166(21):2322-8. doi:10.1001/archinte.166.21.2322
36. Wang TJ, Parise H, Levy D, et al. Obesity and the risk of new-onset atrial fibrillation. *JAMA*. Nov 24 2004;292(20):2471-7. doi:10.1001/jama.292.20.2471
37. Glover BM, Hong KL, Dagres N, et al. Impact of body mass index on the outcome of catheter ablation of atrial fibrillation. *Heart*. 02 2019;105(3):244-250. doi:10.1136/heartjnl-2018-313490
38. Strasser B, Spreitzer A, Haber P. Fat loss depends on energy deficit only, independently of the method for weight loss. *Ann Nutr Metab*. 2007;51(5):428-32. doi:10.1159/000111162
39. Sacks FM, Bray GA, Carey VJ, et al. Comparison of weight-loss diets with different compositions of fat, protein, and carbohydrates. *N Engl J Med*. Feb 26 2009;360(9):859-73. doi:10.1056/NEJMoa0804748
40. Lee HJ, Choi EK, Han KD, et al. Bodyweight fluctuation is associated with increased risk of incident atrial fibrillation. *Heart Rhythm*. 03 2020;17(3):365-371. doi:10.1016/j.hrthm.2019.09.029
41. Hu YF, Chen YJ, Lin YJ, Chen SA. Inflammation and the pathogenesis of atrial fibrillation. *Nat Rev Cardiol*. Apr 2015;12(4):230-43. doi:10.1038/nrcardio.2015.2
42. Byrd DA, Judd SE, Flanders WD, Hartman TJ, Fedirko V, Bostick RM. Development and Validation of Novel Dietary and Lifestyle Inflammation Scores. *J Nutr*. 12 01 2019;149(12):2206-2218. doi:10.1093/jn/nxz165

43. Abed HS, Wittert GA, Leong DP, et al. Effect of weight reduction and cardiometabolic risk factor management on symptom burden and severity in patients with atrial fibrillation: a randomized clinical trial. *JAMA*. Nov 20 2013;310(19):2050-60. doi:10.1001/jama.2013.280521
44. Fernández-Lázaro CI, Ruiz-Canela M, Martínez-González M. Deep dive to the secrets of the PREDIMED trial. *Curr Opin Lipidol*. 02 01 2021;32(1):62-69. doi:10.1097/MOL.0000000000000731
45. Estruch R, Ros E, Salas-Salvadó J, et al. Primary Prevention of Cardiovascular Disease with a Mediterranean Diet Supplemented with Extra-Virgin Olive Oil or Nuts. *N Engl J Med*. Jun 21 2018;378(25):e34. doi:10.1056/NEJMoa1800389
46. Martínez-González M, Toledo E, Arós F, et al. Extravirgin olive oil consumption reduces risk of atrial fibrillation: the PREDIMED (Prevención con Dieta Mediterránea) trial. *Circulation*. Jul 01 2014;130(1):18-26. doi:10.1161/CIRCULATIONAHA.113.006921
47. Salas-Salvadó J, Bulló M, Estruch R, et al. Prevention of diabetes with Mediterranean diets: a subgroup analysis of a randomized trial. *Ann Intern Med*. Jan 07 2014;160(1):1-10. doi:10.7326/M13-1725
48. Ruiz-Canela M, Estruch R, Corella D, Salas-Salvadó J, Martínez-González MA. Association of Mediterranean diet with peripheral artery disease: the PREDIMED randomized trial. *JAMA*. 2014 Jan 22-29 2014;311(4):415-417. doi:10.1001/jama.2013.280618
49. Toledo E, Salas-Salvadó J, Donat-Vargas C, et al. Mediterranean Diet and Invasive Breast Cancer Risk Among Women at High Cardiovascular Risk in the PREDIMED Trial: A Randomized Clinical Trial. *JAMA Intern Med*. Nov 2015;175(11):1752-1760. doi:10.1001/jamainternmed.2015.4838
50. Papadaki A, Martínez-González M, Alonso-Gómez A, et al. Mediterranean diet and risk of heart failure: results from the PREDIMED randomized controlled trial. *Eur J Heart Fail*. 09 2017;19(9):1179-1185. doi:10.1002/ejhf.750
51. Angeloni C, Malaguti M, Barbalace MC, Hrelia S. Bioactivity of Olive Oil Phenols in Neuroprotection. *Int J Mol Sci*. Oct 25 2017;18(11)doi:10.3390/ijms18112230
52. Elliott AD, Linz D, Verdicchio CV, Sanders P. Exercise and Atrial Fibrillation: Prevention or Causation? *Heart Lung Circ*. Sep 2018;27(9):1078-1085. doi:10.1016/j.hlc.2018.04.296
53. Northey JM, Rattray B, Pumpa KL, et al. Can the intensity of physical activity be accurately measured in older adults using questionnaires? *J Sci Med Sport*. Jul 2019;22(7):803-807. doi:10.1016/j.jsams.2019.01.004
54. Khurshid S, Weng LC, Al-Alusi MA, et al. Accelerometer-derived physical activity and risk of atrial fibrillation. *Eur Heart J*. 07 01 2021;42(25):2472-2483. doi:10.1093/eurheartj/ehab250
55. Jetté M, Sidney K, Blümchen G. Metabolic equivalents (METS) in exercise testing, exercise prescription, and evaluation of functional capacity. *Clin Cardiol*. Aug 1990;13(8):555-65. doi:10.1002/clc.4960130809
56. Kaminski J. Metabolic Equivalents for Weight Loss: What Are They & How to Calculate Them. National Academy of Sports Medicine. Accessed November 7, 2022, 2022. https://blog.nasm.org/metabolic-equivalents-for-weight-loss
57. Coelho-Ravagnani CdF, Melo FCL, Ravagnani FC, Burini FHP, Burini RC. Estimation of metabolic equivalent (MET) of an exercise protocol based on indirect calorimetry. *Revista Brasileira de Medicina do Esporte*. 2013;19:134-138.
58. Soliman EZ, Rahman AF, Zhang ZM, et al. Effect of Intensive Blood Pressure Lowering on the Risk of Atrial Fibrillation. *Hypertension*. 06 2020;75(6):1491-1496. doi:10.1161/HYPERTENSIONAHA.120.14766
59. He FJ, MacGregor GA. Reducing population salt intake worldwide: from evidence to implementation. *Prog Cardiovasc Dis*. 2010 Mar-Apr 2010;52(5):363-82. doi:10.1016/j.pcad.2009.12.006
60. Singer DE, Nathan DM, Anderson KM, Wilson PW, Evans JC. Association of HbA1c with prevalent cardiovascular disease in the original cohort of the Framingham Heart Study. *Diabetes*. Feb 1992;41(2):202-8. doi:10.2337/diab.41.2.202
61. Steven S, Hollingsworth KG, Al-Mrabeh A, et al. Very Low-Calorie Diet and 6 Months of Weight Stability in Type 2 Diabetes: Pathophysiological Changes in Responders and Nonresponders. *Diabetes Care*. May 2016;39(5):808-15. doi:10.2337/dc15-1942
62. Ostropolets A, Elias PA, Reyes MV, et al. Metformin Is Associated With a Lower Risk of Atrial Fibrillation and Ventricular Arrhythmias Compared With Sulfonylureas: An Observational Study. *Circ Arrhythm Electrophysiol*. 03 2021;14(3):e009115. doi:10.1161/CIRCEP.120.009115

63. Clinic C. Give Your Good Cholesterol a Boost. Accessed October 20, 2022, 2022. https://health.clevelandclinic.org/hdl-is-it-possible-to-raise-your-good-cholesterol-2/
64. Clinic C. Triglycerides. Accessed October 20, 2022, 2022. https://my.clevelandclinic.org/health/articles/11117-triglycerides
65. Fang WT, Li HJ, Zhang H, Jiang S. The role of statin therapy in the prevention of atrial fibrillation: a meta-analysis of randomized controlled trials. *Br J Clin Pharmacol*. Nov 2012;74(5):744-56. doi:10.1111/j.1365-2125.2012.04258.x
66. Sattar N, Preiss D, Murray HM, et al. Statins and risk of incident diabetes: a collaborative meta-analysis of randomised statin trials. *Lancet*. Feb 27 2010;375(9716):735-42. doi:10.1016/S0140-6736(09)61965-6
67. Abramson J. Statins in Persons at Low Risk of Cardiovascular Disease. *Am Fam Physician*. Nov 01 2017;96(9):Online.
68. Kennedy C, Köller Y, Surkova E. Effect of Coenzyme Q10 on statin-associated myalgia and adherence to statin therapy: A systematic review and meta-analysis. *Atherosclerosis*. 04 2020;299:1-8. doi:10.1016/j.atherosclerosis.2020.03.006
69. Phillips TG. Looking at the benefit of statins from a different perspective. *Am Fam Physician*. Oct 01 2010;82(7):741.
70. Larsson SC, Drca N, Wolk A. Alcohol consumption and risk of atrial fibrillation: a prospective study and dose-response meta-analysis. *J Am Coll Cardiol*. Jul 22 2014;64(3):281-9. doi:10.1016/j.jacc.2014.03.048
71. Champagne B, Arora M, ElSayed A, Beger B, Naidoo P, Shilton T. The impact of alcohol consumption on cardiovascular health: myths and measures. World Heart Federation. https://world-heart-federation.org/wp-content/uploads/WHF-Policy-Brief-Alcohol.pdf
72. Baan R, Straif K, Grosse Y, et al. Carcinogenicity of alcoholic beverages. *Lancet Oncol*. Apr 2007;8(4):292-3. doi:10.1016/s1470-2045(07)70099-2
73. Hasin DS, Stinson FS, Ogburn E, Grant BF. Prevalence, correlates, disability, and comorbidity of DSM-IV alcohol abuse and dependence in the United States: results from the National Epidemiologic Survey on Alcohol and Related Conditions. *Arch Gen Psychiatry*. Jul 2007;64(7):830-42. doi:10.1001/archpsyc.64.7.830
74. Rusyn I, Bataller R. Alcohol and toxicity. *J Hepatol*. Aug 2013;59(2):387-8. doi:10.1016/j.jhep.2013.01.035
75. Organization WH. *Global status report on alcohol and health 2018*. World Health Organization; 2019.
76. Fein AS, Shvilkin A, Shah D, et al. Treatment of obstructive sleep apnea reduces the risk of atrial fibrillation recurrence after catheter ablation. *J Am Coll Cardiol*. Jul 23 2013;62(4):300-5. doi:10.1016/j.jacc.2013.03.052
77. Young T, Palta M, Dempsey J, Peppard PE, Nieto FJ, Hla KM. Burden of sleep apnea: rationale, design, and major findings of the Wisconsin Sleep Cohort study. *WMJ*. Aug 2009;108(5):246-9.
78. Drager LF, Togeiro SM, Polotsky VY, Lorenzi-Filho G. Obstructive sleep apnea: a cardiometabolic risk in obesity and the metabolic syndrome. *J Am Coll Cardiol*. Aug 13 2013;62(7):569-76. doi:10.1016/j.jacc.2013.05.045
79. Kuna ST, Reboussin DM, Strotmeyer ES, et al. Effects of Weight Loss on Obstructive Sleep Apnea Severity. Ten-Year Results of the Sleep AHEAD Study. *Am J Respir Crit Care Med*. 01 15 2021;203(2):221-229. doi:10.1164/rccm.201912-2511OC
80. Spiegel K, Tasali E, Penev P, Van Cauter E. Brief communication: Sleep curtailment in healthy young men is associated with decreased leptin levels, elevated ghrelin levels, and increased hunger and appetite. *Ann Intern Med*. Dec 07 2004;141(11):846-50. doi:10.7326/0003-4819-141-11-200412070-00008
81. Heeringa J, Kors JA, Hofman A, van Rooij FJ, Witteman JC. Cigarette smoking and risk of atrial fibrillation: the Rotterdam Study. *Am Heart J*. Dec 2008;156(6):1163-9. doi:10.1016/j.ahj.2008.08.003
82. Hartmann-Boyce J, Chepkin SC, Ye W, Bullen C, Lancaster T. Nicotine replacement therapy versus control for smoking cessation. *Cochrane Database Syst Rev*. 05 31 2018;5:CD000146. doi:10.1002/14651858.CD000146.pub5
83. Howes S, Hartmann-Boyce J, Livingstone-Banks J, Hong B, Lindson N. Antidepressants for smoking cessation. *Cochrane Database Syst Rev*. 04 22 2020;4:CD000031. doi:10.1002/14651858.CD000031.pub5

84. Hughes JR, Stead LF, Hartmann-Boyce J, Cahill K, Lancaster T. Antidepressants for smoking cessation. *Cochrane Database Syst Rev*. Jan 08 2014;(1):CD000031. doi:10.1002/14651858.CD000031.pub4
85. Patnode CD, Henderson JT, Coppola EL, Melnikow J, Durbin S, Thomas RG. Interventions for Tobacco Cessation in Adults, Including Pregnant Persons: Updated Evidence Report and Systematic Review for the US Preventive Services Task Force. *JAMA*. 01 19 2021;325(3):280-298. doi:10.1001/jama.2020.23541
86. Cahill K, Lindson-Hawley N, Thomas KH, Fanshawe TR, Lancaster T. Nicotine receptor partial agonists for smoking cessation. *Cochrane Database Syst Rev*. May 09 2016;(5):CD006103. doi:10.1002/14651858.CD006103.pub7
87. Lindson N, Chepkin SC, Ye W, Fanshawe TR, Bullen C, Hartmann-Boyce J. Different doses, durations and modes of delivery of nicotine replacement therapy for smoking cessation. *Cochrane Database Syst Rev*. 04 18 2019;4:CD013308. doi:10.1002/14651858.CD013308
88. Hollands GJ, Naughton F, Farley A, Lindson N, Aveyard P. Interventions to increase adherence to medications for tobacco dependence. *Cochrane Database Syst Rev*. 08 16 2019;8:CD009164. doi:10.1002/14651858.CD009164.pub3
89. Ussher MH, Faulkner GEJ, Angus K, Hartmann-Boyce J, Taylor AH. Exercise interventions for smoking cessation. *Cochrane Database Syst Rev*. 10 30 2019;2019(10)doi:10.1002/14651858.CD002295.pub6
90. DiNicolantonio JJ, O'Keefe JH, Wilson W. Subclinical magnesium deficiency: a principal driver of cardiovascular disease and a public health crisis. *Open Heart*. 2018 2018;5(1):e000668. doi:10.1136/openhrt-2017-000668
91. Torshin IY, Gromova OA, Kalacheva AG, Oshchepkova EV, Martynov AI. [Meta-analysis of clinical trials of cardiovascular effects of magnesium orotate]. *Ter Arkh*. 2015;87(6):88-97. doi:10.17116/terarkh201587688-97
92. Alonso A, Rooney MR, Chen LY, et al. Circulating electrolytes and the prevalence of atrial fibrillation and supraventricular ectopy: The Atherosclerosis Risk in Communities (ARIC) study. *Nutr Metab Cardiovasc Dis*. 06 25 2020;30(7):1121-1129. doi:10.1016/j.numecd.2020.03.010
93. Khan AM, Lubitz SA, Sullivan LM, et al. Low serum magnesium and the development of atrial fibrillation in the community: the Framingham Heart Study. *Circulation*. Jan 01 2013;127(1):33-8. doi:10.1161/CIRCULATIONAHA.111.082511
94. Workinger JL, Doyle RP, Bortz J. Challenges in the Diagnosis of Magnesium Status. *Nutrients*. Sep 01 2018;10(9)doi:10.3390/nu10091202
95. Falco CN, Grupi C, Sosa E, et al. Successful improvement of frequency and symptoms of premature complexes after oral magnesium administration. *Arq Bras Cardiol*. Jun 2012;98(6):480-7. doi:10.1590/s0066-782x2012005000043
96. The Nutrition Source: Magnesium. Harvard T.H. Chan School of Public Health. Accessed December 13, 2021, 2021. https://www.hsph.harvard.edu/nutritionsource/magnesium/
97. Veronese N, Pizzol D, Smith L, Dominguez LJ, Barbagallo M. Effect of Magnesium Supplementation on Inflammatory Parameters: A Meta-Analysis of Randomized Controlled Trials. *Nutrients*. Feb 05 2022;14(3)doi:10.3390/nu14030679
98. Kass L, Weekes J, Carpenter L. Effect of magnesium supplementation on blood pressure: a meta-analysis. *Eur J Clin Nutr*. Apr 2012;66(4):411-8. doi:10.1038/ejcn.2012.4
99. Joo Suk O. Paradoxical hypomagnesemia caused by excessive ingestion of magnesium hydroxide. *Am J Emerg Med*. Sep 2008;26(7):837.e1-2. doi:10.1016/j.ajem.2008.01.030
100. Blancquaert L, Vervaet C, Derave W. Predicting and Testing Bioavailability of Magnesium Supplements. *Nutrients*. Jul 20 2019;11(7)doi:10.3390/nu11071663
101. Puścion-Jakubik A, Bartosiewicz N, Socha K. Is the Magnesium Content in Food Supplements Consistent with the Manufacturers' Declarations? *Nutrients*. Sep 28 2021;13(10)doi:10.3390/nu13103416
102. Cogswell ME, Zhang Z, Carriquiry AL, et al. Sodium and potassium intakes among US adults: NHANES 2003-2008. *Am J Clin Nutr*. Sep 2012;96(3):647-57. doi:10.3945/ajcn.112.034413
103. The Nutrition Source: Potassium. Harvard T.H. Chan School of Public Health. Accessed February 8, 2022, https://www.hsph.harvard.edu/nutritionsource/potassium/
104. Potassium Fact Sheet for Health Professionals. National Institutes of Health. Accessed November 10, 2022, https://ods.od.nih.gov/factsheets/Potassium-HealthProfessional/#en27

105. Krijthe BP, Heeringa J, Kors JA, et al. Serum potassium levels and the risk of atrial fibrillation: the Rotterdam Study. *Int J Cardiol*. Oct 15 2013;168(6):5411-5. doi:10.1016/j.ijcard.2013.08.048
106. D'Elia L, Barba G, Cappuccio FP, Strazzullo P. Potassium intake, stroke, and cardiovascular disease a meta-analysis of prospective studies. *J Am Coll Cardiol*. Mar 08 2011;57(10):1210-9. doi:10.1016/j.jacc.2010.09.070
107. CFR - Code of Federal Regulations Title 21. US Food and Drug Administration. Accessed November 10, 2022, 2022. https://www.accessdata.fda.gov/scripts/cdrh/cfdocs/cfcfr/CFRSearch.cfm?fr=201.306
108. Papathanasiou KA, Giotaki SG, Vrachatis DA, et al. Molecular Insights in Atrial Fibrillation Pathogenesis and Therapeutics: A Narrative Review. *Diagnostics (Basel)*. Aug 31 2021;11(9)doi:10.3390/diagnostics11091584
109. Pool L, Wijdeveld LFJM, de Groot NMS, Brundel BJJM. The Role of Mitochondrial Dysfunction in Atrial Fibrillation: Translation to Druggable Target and Biomarker Discovery. *Int J Mol Sci*. Aug 06 2021;22(16)doi:10.3390/ijms22168463
110. Martelli A, Testai L, Colletti A, Cicero AFG. Coenzyme Q. *Antioxidants (Basel)*. Apr 22 2020;9(4)doi:10.3390/antiox9040341
111. Mantle D, Heaton RA, Hargreaves IP. Coenzyme Q10 and Immune Function: An Overview. *Antioxidants (Basel)*. May 11 2021;10(5)doi:10.3390/antiox10050759
112. Hu YF, Wu CH, Lai TC, et al. ALDH2 deficiency induces atrial fibrillation through dysregulated cardiac sodium channel and mitochondrial bioenergetics: A multi-omics analysis. *Biochim Biophys Acta Mol Basis Dis*. 05 01 2021;1867(5):166088. doi:10.1016/j.bbadis.2021.166088
113. Zhao Q, Kebbati AH, Zhang Y, Tang Y, Okello E, Huang C. Effect of coenzyme Q10 on the incidence of atrial fibrillation in patients with heart failure. *J Investig Med*. Jun 2015;63(5):735-9. doi:10.1097/JIM.0000000000000202
114. de Frutos F, Gea A, Hernandez-Estefania R, Rabago G. Prophylactic treatment with coenzyme Q10 in patients undergoing cardiac surgery: could an antioxidant reduce complications? A systematic review and meta-analysis. *Interact Cardiovasc Thorac Surg*. Feb 2015;20(2):254-9. doi:10.1093/icvts/ivu334
115. Hidaka T, Fujii K, Funahashi I, Fukutomi N, Hosoe K. Safety assessment of coenzyme Q10 (CoQ10). *Biofactors*. 2008;32(1-4):199-208. doi:10.1002/biof.5520320124
116. Ho MJ, Li EC, Wright JM. Blood pressure lowering efficacy of coenzyme Q10 for primary hypertension. *Cochrane Database Syst Rev*. Mar 03 2016;3:CD007435. doi:10.1002/14651858.CD007435.pub3
117. Liu DC, Yan JJ, Wang YN, et al. Low-dose green tea intake reduces incidence of atrial fibrillation in a Chinese population. *Oncotarget*. Dec 20 2016;7(51):85592-85602. doi:10.18632/oncotarget.12243
118. Zhu J, Zhang X, Li L, Su G. Protective effects of epigallocatechin-3 gallate on atrial electrical and structural remodeling in a rabbit rapid atrial pacing model. *Cell Biochem Biophys*. Mar 2015;71(2):897-903. doi:10.1007/s12013-014-0280-2
119. Liu G, Mi XN, Zheng XX, Xu YL, Lu J, Huang XH. Effects of tea intake on blood pressure: a meta-analysis of randomised controlled trials. *Br J Nutr*. Oct 14 2014;112(7):1043-54. doi:10.1017/S0007114514001731
120. Kotronia E, Brown H, Papacosta AO, et al. Oral health and all-cause, cardiovascular disease, and respiratory mortality in older people in the UK and USA. *Sci Rep*. 08 12 2021;11(1):16452. doi:10.1038/s41598-021-95865-z
121. Chang Y, Woo HG, Park J, Lee JS, Song TJ. Improved oral hygiene care is associated with decreased risk of occurrence for atrial fibrillation and heart failure: A nationwide population-based cohort study. *Eur J Prev Cardiol*. 11 2020;27(17):1835-1845. doi:10.1177/2047487319886018
122. Chen SJ, Liu CJ, Chao TF, et al. Dental scaling and atrial fibrillation: a nationwide cohort study. *Int J Cardiol*. Oct 03 2013;168(3):2300-3. doi:10.1016/j.ijcard.2013.01.192
123. Illinois DDo. Delta Dental of Illinois 2014 Oral Health and Well-Being Survey. 2015.
124. Pitchika V, Pink C, Völzke H, Welk A, Kocher T, Holtfreter B. Long-term impact of powered toothbrush on oral health: 11-year cohort study. *J Clin Periodontol*. 07 2019;46(7):713-722. doi:10.1111/jcpe.13126
125. Petti S, Scully C. Polyphenols, oral health and disease: A review. *J Dent*. Jun 2009;37(6):413-23. doi:10.1016/j.jdent.2009.02.003
126. Mirabelli M, Chiefari E, Arcidiacono B, et al. Mediterranean Diet Nutrients to Turn the Tide against Insulin Resistance and Related Diseases. *Nutrients*. Apr 12 2020;12(4)doi:10.3390/nu12041066

127. Maruyama T, Fukata M, Akashi K. Association of atrial fibrillation and gastroesophageal reflux disease: Natural and therapeutic linkage of the two common diseases. *J Arrhythm*. Feb 2019;35(1):43-51. doi:10.1002/joa3.12125
128. Malik A, Best K, Singh S, Jaggon KS, Michael M. Hiatal Hernia: A Possible Trigger for Atrial Fibrillation. *Cureus*. Oct 2021;13(10):e18857. doi:10.7759/cureus.18857
129. Xu L, Zhang Y, Xie J, Liu Y. Association between gastroesophageal reflux disease and atrial fibrillation: a systematic review and meta-analysis. *Rev Esp Enferm Dig*. Nov 2019;111(11):874-879. doi:10.17235/reed.2019.5389/2017
130. LiverTox. Clinical and Research Information on Drug-Induced Liver Injury: Proton Pump Inhibitors. Internet. National Institute of Diabetes and Digestive and Kidney Diseases. Accessed July 19, 2022, 2022. https://www.ncbi.nlm.nih.gov/books/NBK547892/
131. Srinutta T, Chewcharat A, Takkavatakarn K, et al. Proton pump inhibitors and hypomagnesemia: A meta-analysis of observational studies. *Medicine (Baltimore)*. Nov 2019;98(44):e17788. doi:10.1097/MD.0000000000017788
132. Essrani R, Mehershahi S, Ravi SJK, et al. Famotidine induced hypomagnesemia leading to hypocalcemia. *Oxf Med Case Reports*. Jan 2020;2020(1):omz133. doi:10.1093/omcr/omz133
133. Newberry C, Lynch K. The role of diet in the development and management of gastroesophageal reflux disease: why we feel the burn. *J Thorac Dis*. Aug 2019;11(Suppl 12):S1594-S1601. doi:10.21037/jtd.2019.06.42
134. Fujiwara Y, Machida A, Watanabe Y, et al. Association between dinner-to-bed time and gastro-esophageal reflux disease. *Am J Gastroenterol*. Dec 2005;100(12):2633-6. doi:10.1111/j.1572-0241.2005.00354.x
135. Mone I, Kraja B, Bregu A, et al. Adherence to a predominantly Mediterranean diet decreases the risk of gastroesophageal reflux disease: a cross-sectional study in a South Eastern European population. *Dis Esophagus*. Oct 2016;29(7):794-800. doi:10.1111/dote.12384
136. Zalvan CH, Hu S, Greenberg B, Geliebter J. A Comparison of Alkaline Water and Mediterranean Diet vs Proton Pump Inhibition for Treatment of Laryngopharyngeal Reflux. *JAMA Otolaryngol Head Neck Surg*. 10 01 2017;143(10):1023-1029. doi:10.1001/jamaoto.2017.1454
137. Carlsen MH, Halvorsen BL, Holte K, et al. The total antioxidant content of more than 3100 foods, beverages, spices, herbs and supplements used worldwide. *Nutr J*. Jan 22 2010;9:3. doi:10.1186/1475-2891-9-3
138. Eastman P. New Research on Antioxidants Shows Surprising Role for Coffee. *Oncology Times*. 2005;27(20):39-40. doi:10.1097/01.cot.0000290968.61298.07
139. Grotto D, Zied E. The Standard American Diet and its relationship to the health status of Americans. *Nutr Clin Pract*. Dec 2010;25(6):603-12. doi:10.1177/0884533610386234
140. Symbols IoMUCoEoF-o-PNRSa. Front-of-Package Nutrition Rating Systems and Symbols: Phase I Report. 2010.
141. Pérez-Jiménez J, Neveu V, Vos F, Scalbert A. Identification of the 100 richest dietary sources of polyphenols: an application of the Phenol-Explorer database. *Eur J Clin Nutr*. Nov 2010;64 Suppl 3:S112-20. doi:10.1038/ejcn.2010.221
142. Akhtar MS, Ramzan A, Ali A, Ahmad M. Effect of Amla fruit (Emblica officinalis Gaertn.) on blood glucose and lipid profile of normal subjects and type 2 diabetic patients. *Int J Food Sci Nutr*. Sep 2011;62(6):609-16. doi:10.3109/09637486.2011.560565
143. Gul M, Liu ZW, Iahtisham-Ul-Haq, et al. Functional and Nutraceutical Significance of Amla (*Phyllanthus emblica* L.): A Review. *Antioxidants (Basel)*. Apr 22 2022;11(5)doi:10.3390/antiox11050816
144. Dolara P, Bigagli E, Collins A. Antioxidant vitamins and mineral supplementation, life span expansion and cancer incidence: a critical commentary. *Eur J Nutr*. Oct 2012;51(7):769-81. doi:10.1007/s00394-012-0389-2
145. Hu X, Yuan L, Wang H, et al. Efficacy and safety of vitamin C for atrial fibrillation after cardiac surgery: A meta-analysis with trial sequential analysis of randomized controlled trials. *Int J Surg*. Jan 2017;37:58-64. doi:10.1016/j.ijsu.2016.12.009
146. Hemilä H. Errors in a meta-analysis on vitamin C and post-operative atrial fibrillation. *Int J Surg*. Apr 2019;64:66. doi:10.1016/j.ijsu.2019.01.025

147. Krittanawong C, Tunhasiriwet A, Wang Z, et al. Is caffeine or coffee consumption a risk for new-onset atrial fibrillation? A systematic review and meta-analysis. *Eur J Prev Cardiol*. Oct 13 2021;28(12):e13-e15. doi:10.1177/2047487320908385
148. Andres S, Pevny S, Ziegenhagen R, et al. Safety Aspects of the Use of Quercetin as a Dietary Supplement. *Mol Nutr Food Res*. 01 2018;62(1)doi:10.1002/mnfr.201700447
149. Corega C, Vaida L, Festila DG, et al. The benefits of Quercitin for dentistry and maxillofacial surgery: a systematic review. *Minerva Stomatol*. Jan 14 2014;
150. Wang H, Jiang W, Hu Y, et al. Quercetin improves atrial fibrillation through inhibiting TGF-β/Smads pathway via promoting MiR-135b expression. *Phytomedicine*. Dec 2021;93:153774. doi:10.1016/j.phymed.2021.153774
151. Tan X, Xian W, Li X, et al. Mechanisms of Quercetin against atrial fibrillation explored by network pharmacology combined with molecular docking and experimental validation. *Sci Rep*. Jun 13 2022;12(1):9777. doi:10.1038/s41598-022-13911-w
152. Hu J, Wang X, Cui X, Kuang W, Li D, Wang J. Quercetin prevents isoprenaline-induced myocardial fibrosis by promoting autophagy via regulating miR-223-3p/FOXO3. *Cell Cycle*. 07 2021;20(13):1253-1269. doi:10.1080/15384101.2021.1932029
153. Hosseini A, Razavi BM, Banach M, Hosseinzadeh H. Quercetin and metabolic syndrome: A review. *Phytother Res*. Oct 2021;35(10):5352-5364. doi:10.1002/ptr.7144
154. Serban MC, Sahebkar A, Zanchetti A, et al. Effects of Quercetin on Blood Pressure: A Systematic Review and Meta-Analysis of Randomized Controlled Trials. *J Am Heart Assoc*. 07 12 2016;5(7)doi:10.1161/JAHA.115.002713
155. Egert S, Bosy-Westphal A, Seiberl J, et al. Quercetin reduces systolic blood pressure and plasma oxidised low-density lipoprotein concentrations in overweight subjects with a high-cardiovascular disease risk phenotype: a double-blinded, placebo-controlled cross-over study. *Br J Nutr*. Oct 2009;102(7):1065-74. doi:10.1017/S0007114509359127
156. Okamoto T. Safety of quercetin for clinical application (Review). *Int J Mol Med*. Aug 2005;16(2):275-8.
157. Cheeseman M. GRAS Notice Inventory-Agency Response Letter GRAS Notice No. GRN 00034. Silver Spring, MD: U.S. Food and Drug Administration; 2010.
158. Administration UFaD. Questions and Answers on Dietary Supplements. College Park, MD: US Food and Drug Administration; 2022.
159. Zuo K, Yin X, Li K, et al. Different Types of Atrial Fibrillation Share Patterns of Gut Microbiota Dysbiosis. *mSphere*. 03 18 2020;5(2)doi:10.1128/mSphere.00071-20
160. Lu D, Zou X, Zhang H. The Relationship Between Atrial Fibrillation and Intestinal Flora With Its Metabolites. *Front Cardiovasc Med*. 2022;9:948755. doi:10.3389/fcvm.2022.948755
161. Kassaian N, Feizi A, Aminorroaya A, Amini M. Probiotic and synbiotic supplementation could improve metabolic syndrome in prediabetic adults: A randomized controlled trial. *Diabetes Metab Syndr*. 2019 Sep - Oct 2019;13(5):2991-2996. doi:10.1016/j.dsx.2018.07.016
162. Quigley EM. Gut bacteria in health and disease. *Gastroenterol Hepatol (N Y)*. Sep 2013;9(9):560-9.
163. Sorrenti V, Ali S, Mancin L, Davinelli S, Paoli A, Scapagnini G. Cocoa Polyphenols and Gut Microbiota Interplay: Bioavailability, Prebiotic Effect, and Impact on Human Health. *Nutrients*. Jun 27 2020;12(7)doi:10.3390/nu12071908
164. Slavin J. Fiber and prebiotics: mechanisms and health benefits. *Nutrients*. Apr 22 2013;5(4):1417-35. doi:10.3390/nu5041417
165. Dimidi E, Cox SR, Rossi M, Whelan K. Fermented Foods: Definitions and Characteristics, Impact on the Gut Microbiota and Effects on Gastrointestinal Health and Disease. *Nutrients*. Aug 05 2019;11(8)doi:10.3390/nu11081806
166. Andersen ZJ, Cramer J, Jørgensen JT, et al. Long-Term Exposure to Road Traffic Noise and Air Pollution, and Incident Atrial Fibrillation in the Danish Nurse Cohort. *Environ Health Perspect*. Aug 2021;129(8):87002. doi:10.1289/EHP8090
167. Kim IS, Yang PS, Lee J, et al. Long-term exposure of fine particulate matter air pollution and incident atrial fibrillation in the general population: A nationwide cohort study. *Int J Cardiol*. 05 15 2019;283:178-183. doi:10.1016/j.ijcard.2018.12.048
168. Vanchiere C, Thirumal R, Hendrani A, et al. Association Between Atrial Fibrillation and Occupational Exposure in Firefighters Based on Self-Reported Survey Data. *J Am Heart Assoc*. Apr 05 2022;11(7):e022543. doi:10.1161/JAHA.121.022543

169. Bräuner EV, Jørgensen JT, Duun-Henriksen AK, et al. Long-term wind turbine noise exposure and the risk of incident atrial fibrillation in the Danish Nurse cohort. *Environ Int*. Sep 2019;130:104915. doi:10.1016/j.envint.2019.104915
170. Torén K, Schiöler L, Söderberg M, Giang KW, Rosengren A. The association between job strain and atrial fibrillation in Swedish men. *Occup Environ Med*. Mar 2015;72(3):177-80. doi:10.1136/oemed-2014-102256
171. Karasek R, Baker D, Marxer F, Ahlbom A, Theorell T. Job decision latitude, job demands, and cardiovascular disease: a prospective study of Swedish men. *Am J Public Health*. Jul 1981;71(7):694-705. doi:10.2105/ajph.71.7.694
172. Eaker ED, Sullivan LM, Kelly-Hayes M, D'Agostino RB, Benjamin EJ. Anger and hostility predict the development of atrial fibrillation in men in the Framingham Offspring Study. *Circulation*. Mar 16 2004;109(10):1267-71. doi:10.1161/01.CIR.0000118535.15205.8F
173. Eaker ED, Sullivan LM, Kelly-Hayes M, D'Agostino RB, Benjamin EJ. Tension and anxiety and the prediction of the 10-year incidence of coronary heart disease, atrial fibrillation, and total mortality: the Framingham Offspring Study. *Psychosom Med*. 2005 Sep-Oct 2005;67(5):692-6. doi:10.1097/01.psy.0000174050.87193.96
174. Lampert R, Jamner L, Burg M, et al. Triggering of symptomatic atrial fibrillation by negative emotion. *J Am Coll Cardiol*. Oct 07 2014;64(14):1533-4. doi:10.1016/j.jacc.2014.07.959
175. Salari-Moghaddam A, Keshteli AH, Afshar H, Esmaillzadeh A, Adibi P. Empirically derived food-based dietary inflammatory index is associated with increased risk of psychological disorders in women. *Nutr Neurosci*. Apr 2021;24(4):260-268. doi:10.1080/1028415X.2019.1621044
176. Li X, Zhou T, Ma H, et al. Healthy Sleep Patterns and Risk of Incident Arrhythmias. *J Am Coll Cardiol*. Sep 21 2021;78(12):1197-1207. doi:10.1016/j.jacc.2021.07.023
177. Wang N, Sun Y, Zhang H, et al. Long-term night shift work is associated with the risk of atrial fibrillation and coronary heart disease. *Eur Heart J*. Oct 21 2021;42(40):4180-4188. doi:10.1093/eurheartj/ehab505
178. Hansson A, Madsen-Härdig B, Olsson SB. Arrhythmia-provoking factors and symptoms at the onset of paroxysmal atrial fibrillation: a study based on interviews with 100 patients seeking hospital assistance. *BMC Cardiovasc Disord*. Aug 03 2004;4:13. doi:10.1186/1471-2261-4-13
179. Andreasen L, Nielsen JB, Olesen MS. Genetic aspects of lone atrial fibrillation: what do we know? *Curr Pharm Des*. 2015;21(5):667-78. doi:10.2174/1381612820666140825143610
180. Khera AV, Emdin CA, Drake I, et al. Genetic Risk, Adherence to a Healthy Lifestyle, and Coronary Disease. *N Engl J Med*. 12 15 2016;375(24):2349-2358. doi:10.1056/NEJMoa1605086

Made in the USA
Monee, IL
05 November 2026

67845294R00044